Inflammatory Bowel Disease and Coeliac Disease in Children

Inflammatory Bowel Disease and Coeliac Disease in Children

EDITED BY

F. Hadziselimovic
B. Herzog
A. Bürgin-Wolff
University of Basel
Switzerland

Proceedings of the International Falk Symposium on Pediatric and Surgical
Gastroenterology held in Basel, Switzerland, November 10–11, 1989

KLUWER ACADEMIC PUBLISHERS
DORDRECHT / BOSTON / LONDON

Distributors

for the United States and Canada: Kluwer Academic Publishers, PO Box 358, Accord Station, Hingham, MA 02018-0358, USA
for all other countries: Kluwer Academic Publishers Group, Distribution Centre, PO Box 322, 3300 AH Dordrecht, The Netherlands

British Library Cataloguing in Publication Data

International Falk Symposium on Pediatric and Surgical
    Gastroenterology (*1989 ; Basel ; Switzerland*)
    Inflammatory bowel disease and coeliac disease in
    children.
    1. Children. Intestines. Diseases
    I. Title   II. Hadziselimovic, F.   III. Herzog, B.
    IV. Bürgin-Wolff, A.
    618.9234

ISBN 0-7462-0125-7

Published in the United Kingdom by Kluwer Academic Publishers, PO Box 55, Lancaster, UK.

Kluwer Academic Publishers BV incorporates the publishing programmes of D. Reidel, Martinus Nijhoff, Dr W. Junk and MTP Press.

Printed in Great Britain by Butler and Tanner Ltd., Frome and London

Contents

Preface   vii

List of Principal Contributors   ix

SECTION I: INFLAMMATORY BOWEL DISEASE

1   Postnatal immunomorphology of the gut
J.-O. Gebbers and J.A. Laissue   3

2   Genetics of inflammatory bowel disease
A.S. Peña   45

3   Special aspects of inflammatory bowel disease in children
B.S. Kirschner   59

4   Evaluation of endoscopic findings in Crohn's disease of
childhood and adolescence
*M. Burdelski, H.-G. Posselt, M. Becker, R.-M. Bertele-Harms,
B. Rodeck, P.-F. Hoyer and P. Schmitz-Moormann*   67

5   Diagnostic imaging in inflammatory bowel disease in paediatric
patients
C.P. Fliegel and F. Hadziselimovic   75

6   Lymphocyte subsets in Crohn's disease
B. Rodeck, M.R. Hadam and M. Burdelski   83

7   Medical treatment of chronic inflammatory bowel disease
H.K. Harms   87

8   Toxic effect of sulphasalazine on prepubertal testes
F. Hadziselimovic, B. Keller, U. Hennes and U. Schaub   99

9   Indications for surgery in inflammatory bowel disease
B. Herzog   117

10   Surgery for inflammatory bowel disease: ulcerative colitis
A. Colodny   121

11   Factors that influence the postoperative recurrence of Crohn's
disease in childhood
A.M. Griffiths   131

12 Psyche and inflammatory bowel disease   137
    G. Stacher

SECTION II: COELIAC DISEASE

13 Management of coeliac disease in children: a personal view
    J.A. Walker-Smith   147

14 Grain prolamins: why immunogenic, how toxic?
    W.T.J.M. Hekkens and M. van Twist-de Graaf   157

15 Class II molecules in coeliac disease
    M.L. Mearin   169

16 The diagnostic significance of gliadin and endomysium
    antibodies in childhood coeliac disease
    A. Bürgin-Wolff, H. Gaze, F. Hadziselimovic, M.J. Lentze and
    D. Nusslé   177

17 Concluding remarks
    F. Hadziselimovic   189

    Index   195

Preface

Despite significant progress in modern gastroenterology, the aetiology of inflammatory bowel disease as well as coeliac disease is still to a great extent unknown and poorly understood.

The principles of treatment – particularly of IBD – emphasize the importance of a combined medical and surgical approach.

This book is the proceedings of an international symposium that brought together workers from many disciplines involved in the treatment of IBD and coeliac disease, and is a useful update on recent advances in paediatric and paediatric–surgical gastroenterology.

F. Hadziselimovic, B. Herzog, A. Bürgin-Wolff

List of Principal Contributors

M. BURDELSKI
Kinderklinik
Medizinische Hochschule Hannover
Postfach 61 01 80
D-3000 Hannover 61
FRG

A. BÜRGIN-WOLFF
Basler Kinderspital
Römergasse 8
CH-4005 Basel
Switzerland

A. H. COLODNY
Harvard Medical School
Division of Urology
The Children's Hospital
300 Longwood Avenue
Boston, MA 02115
USA

C. P. FLIEGEL
Department of Radiology
Basler Kinderspital
Römergasse 8
CH-4005 Basel
Switzerland

J.-O. GEBBERS
Institute of Pathology
Kantonsspital
CH-6000 Luzern 16
Switzerland

A. M. GRIFFITHS
Division of Gastroenterology
Hospital for Sick Children
555 University Avenue
Toronto
Ontario M5G 1X8
Canada

F. HADZISELIMOVIC
Department of Gastroenterology
Basler Kinderspital
Römergasse 8
CH-4005 Basel
Switzerland

H. K. HARMS
Dr. V. Hauner'sches Kinderspital
Lindwurmstrasse 4
D-8000 Munich 2
FRG

W. T. J. HEKKENS
Department of Physiology
Faculty of Medicine
University of Leiden
Wassenaarseweg 62
PO Box 9604
NL-2300 RC Leiden
The Netherlands

B. HERZOG
Pediatric Surgery
Basler Kinderspital
Römergasse 8
CH-4005 Basel
Switzerland

B. S. KIRSCHNER
Wyler Children's Hospital
5825 S. Maryland Avenue
Chicago, IL 60637
USA

M. L. MEARIN
Department of Pediatrics
University Hospital Leiden
PO BOx 9600
NL-2300 RC Leiden
The Netherlands

ix

A. S. PEÑA
Department Gastroenterology
University Hospital Leiden
PO Box 9600
NL-2300 RC Leiden
The Netherlands

B. RODECK
Kinderklinik
Medizinische Hochschule Hannover
Postfach 61 01 80
D-3000 Hannover 61
FRG

G. STACHER
Allgemeines Krankenhaus der Stadt Wien
Psychophysiology Laboratory
Währinger Gürtel 18–20
A-1090 Vienna
Austria

J. A. WALKER-SMITH
Academic Department of Paediatric
  Gastroenterology
Queen Elizabeth Hospital for Children
Hackney Road
London, E2 8PS
UK

Section I
Inflammatory Bowel
Disease

1
Postnatal immunomorphology of the gut

J.-O. GEBBERS and J.A. LAISSUE

SUMMARY

The intestine is richly populated with lymphoid tissue capable of initiating and affecting a wide variety of immunological reactions. These reactions have consequences not only for the gut itself but for the body in general, and have established the importance of the *gut as an immunologic organ.*

Among the outer and inner surfaces of our body, the 200–300 m^2 of the gut contrast with the 2 m^2 of the skin, and the 80 m^2 of the lung. At the inner surface of the intestine, our organism contacts intimately bacteria, parasites, enzymes, toxins, a wide variety of dietary substances and their breakdown products.

The essential barrier against the permanent antigenic burden is the mucosa. Its integrity depends on the continual replication, maturation, and metabolism of its constituents. Additional defense functions are exerted by the mucus, lysozyme, phagocytes, other cells, humoral factors and biological response modifiers involved in inflammatory and immune reactions.

Some of these factors are being produced very close to the surface at which they act. The sum of the mechanical, humoral, cellular, immunologic and non-immunologic defense factors of the intestinal mucosa constitutes the *mucosal block.*

However, the block is not complete. Rather, a continuous antigenic uptake through the epithelial layer takes place. The specialized structures of Peyer's patches, solitary lymphatic follicles, appendix vermiformis and their associated epithelium allow a controlled *antigen uptake* (sampling). Because of the heavy antigenic load, the intestine can be described as the most important *immunologic contact organ* of our body. The antigens may give rise to local and systemic immune reactions with antibody production *or* the suppression of systemic immunologic responses to ingested antigens (*oral tolerance*).

Little is known about the *development of the human gut-associated* lymphoid tissue (GALT) after birth and its maintenance during life. We have studied the parenchyma of the human appendix vermiformis, a GALT organ, measuring and counting lymphatic follicles and germinal centres in 190 appendices which had been removed 'incidentally' from persons 1 day to 89 years old. We have also counted the mucosal plasma cells (with IgA, IgG, IgM and IgE). In the first two weeks of postnatal life, the appendix contains no mature plasma cells and very few lymphatic follicles. Germinal centres are not seen before the 4th week of life and are preceded by mature plasma cells, mainly with IgA and IgM; in the first two months, IgM cells prevail.

The adult vermiform appendix harbours a higher proportion of plasma cells with IgG (30%) than the other intestinal mucosa (5%). About 60% of plasma cells contain IgA, and 10% IgM. The concentration of mucosal plasma cells remains constant until old age, whereas lymphatic follicles and germinal centres decrease only slightly until the 9th decade of life.

The newborn lacks the protection due to intestinal secretory IgA during the first two weeks. Our findings contrast with the reported involution with age of the lymphatic tissue in other organs and support the view that the structure and presumably function of the GALT differ from those of extraintestinal lymphatic tissue.

ANTIGENIC BURDEN OF THE GUT

The antigenic burden of the intestinal tract is heavy. Bacteria, viruses, parasites, toxins, enzymes and a host of dietary substances and their breakdown products intimately contact the mammalian organism at the intestinal interface.

There are many *bacteria* in the oral cavity and pharynx, but virtually none in the oesophagus and stomach. In the intestine, the bacterial counts rise progressively from 10^2 to 10^3 organisms per millilitre in the proximal small bowel[1] to approximately 10^{12} (Figure 1). Over one-half of the dry faecal mass was found to consist of microbial cells. Estimates based upon intestinal content and the population levels of bacteria indicated that as many as 10^{14} live in the gut[3]. This means that the number of bacterial cells in our gut is 10 times larger than the estimated number of cells in our body.

One important way the normal microflora affects the organism is to stimulate and enhance its defensive responses. Those influences begin early in postnatal life as the neonatal host matures. They persist throughout life unless the flora is altered by drugs or physiological changes. Immediately after birth the healthy human acquires micro-organisms in its gastrointestinal canal as bacteria start to appear in faeces within 24 hours after birth. An indigenous (autochthonous) microbiota develops soon after birth in a proposed succession of about four periods of time characterized by the bacterial populations that differ in composition and quantity[4]. This development may be influenced by caesarean section, preterm birth, antimicrobial treatment, and the type of feeding (breast milk versus fomula)[5].

Because of a slow transit of intestinal contents, the large bowel is heavily exposed to bacterial and other antigenic substances; it can be considered as the main antigenic contact organ of our organism (Figure 2) .

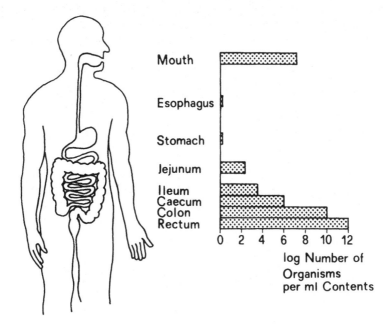

Figure 1 Bacterial counts in different regions of the gastrointestinal tract in normal individuals

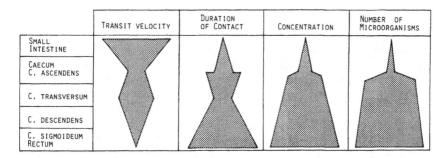

Figure 2 Parameters of the transit of intestinal contents in different regions of the gut (from reference 172)

THE MUCOSAL BLOCK

The essential barrier against the permanent antigenic burden is the mucosa. Although it prevents penetration of potentially noxious agents, its main function is to allow exchange of substances between the gut lumen and the 'milieu intérieur' of the body. The lamina epithelialis mucosae with its rapid cell turnover, the mucus and lysozyme of Paneth cells are important defense mechanisms. The intestine is also equipped with an extensive local immune apparatus that functions fairly independently from the systemic immune mechanisms. The mechanical, humoral, cellular, immunologic, and non-immunologic defense factors in the intestinal mucosa constitute together the mucosal block (Figure 3).

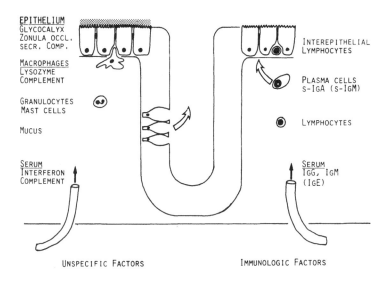

Figure 3   The mucosal block as the sum of unspecific and immunologic barriers of the gut mucosa

However, this block is not absolute. Antigens are continuously taken up through the epithelial layer. The resulting local or systemic immune reactions are twofold: secretion of antibodies, mainly of IgA class, or suppression of systemic immunologic responses to ingested antigens[6] (oral tolerance). The specialized structures of Peyer's patches, solitary lymph follicles and appendix vermiformis allow a controlled uptake (sampling) of antigenic substances. Epithelial cells and their products are essential participants in both initial and final stages of reactivity to foreign materials. They play a role in antigen exclusion, transport of antigens from the lumen, bidirectional transport, degradation of antigens, antigen presentation and antibody secretion[7].

Mucus

The mucus layer, an epithelial product, forms the outer barrier. Mucins are complex hydrated gels composed of a variable group of glycoproteins. The physicochemical properties of the mucus secreted by the goblet cells[8] are ideal for the task of covering, lubricating and protecting a constantly moving surface[9]. The mucus interacts with other secretory products of the intestinal mucosa, such as lysozyme and immunoglobulin A (IgA)[10] (Figure 4). Immunologic events may influence the secretion of mucus[11-13].

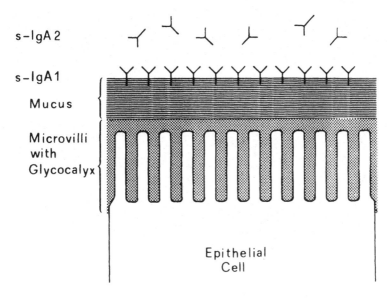

s-IgA 2

s-IgA 1

Mucus

Microvilli with Glycocalyx

Epithelial Cell

Figure 4 Interaction of the intestinal mucus with secretory IgA (hypothesis)

Epithelium: structures

The mucosa of the intestine covers an area[14] of about 200–300 m[2]. This large *surface* warrants an optimal contact for absorption between nutrients and the mucosa. The plicae circulares (Kerckring's folds), the villi intestinales, the glandulae intestinales (crypts of Lieberkühn) (Figure 5) and the microvilli (Figure 6) increase the inner surface of the otherwise smooth tubular small intestine by a factor of 600. The mucosa membrane of the colon has many transverse grooves at distances varying from 0.6 mm to 2 mm (Figure 5). The villi of the small intestine and the colonic 'surface' epithelium absorb intestinal contents, whereas the crypts secrete various substances and replace desquamated cells.

The *columnar villous and colonic surface epithelium* consists of principal cells (enterocytes) and few goblet cells. The polarity of the enterocytes is essential for transepithelial bidirectional transport. The basolateral surface takes up nutrients and also receives hormonal and other signals from the organism. Intercellular spaces in the basal parts of this epithelial layer are important for the absorptive and secretory functions of these cells.

The *brush (or striated) border* at the apical pole of the principal cell consists of 1500 to 3000 microvilli per cell (Figure 6). These finger-like

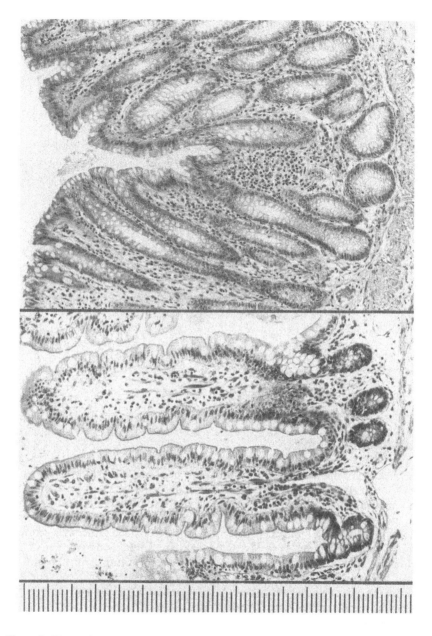

Figure 5 Photomicrographs of the human intestinal mucosa. Bottom: jejunal mucosa with a continuous sheet of simple epithelium which covers the connective tissue of the lamina propria. The crypts rest on the muscularis mucosae, the thin layer of smooth muscle that separates the mucosa from the submucosa below. Note that the crypts are less than one third the length of the finger-shaped villi. Top: colonic mucosa with long crypts of Lieberkühn around a transverse groove. The distance between two marks at the bottom margin is equivalent to 0.2 mm

projections of the cell membrane increase the surface area of the mucosa by a factor of 15 to 25. The microvilli contain a cytoskeleton[15] with myosin, actin and tropomyosin[16]. They can move actively[17].

Filaments synthesized by the epithelium coat its microvillous and intermicrovillous membrane and radiate into the lumen. This *glycocalyx* or fuzzy coat consists of acid glycosoaminoglycans and glycoproteins[18]. The glycocalyx probably increases the absorptive (and digestive?) surface and is an effective barrier to large particles, such as bacteria and fat droplets[18] (Figure 6).

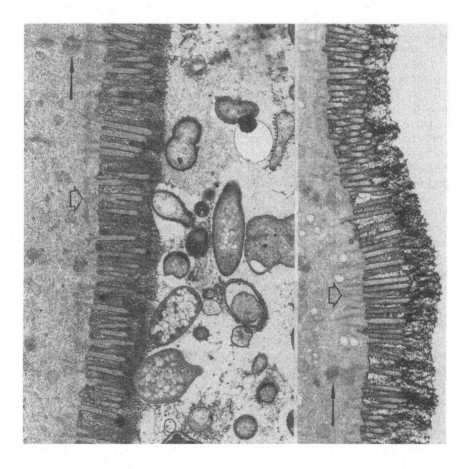

Figure 6 Electron micrograph of human intestinal epithelia with microvilli representing finger-like projections of the apical cell membrane, whose area is markedly increased by them. Bundles of filaments within the microvilli extend the entire length of them and reach into the terminal web (open arrows). Thin filaments which extend from this microvillous membrane into the lumen constitute the glycocalyx (fuzzy coat), a barrier which prevents bacterial contact to the microvillous membrane (bottom). The cell membranes of adjacent cells are joined together just below the surface by the junctional complex (arrows). Ruthenium red ×17700

The epithelial cells are connected by a *junctional complex* which consists of: (a) the most apical zonula occludens (tight junction); (b) the zonula adherens (the underlying intermediate junction); and (c) the macula adherens (desmosomes). The tight junction is located at the base of the brush border (Figure 6). It ties the epithelial cells together and seals epithelial interstices, acting as a diffusion barrier to large molecules, such as haemoglobin, and perhaps also to small molecules, and even to water. The intermediate junction and desmosomes probably tie the cells together.

The *crypt epithelium* is made up of five cell types: goblet cells (Figure 7), differentiated and undifferentiated cells, enterochromaffin cells and, in the small intestine, the caecum and the appendix, the Paneth cells. The cytoplasmic granules of the goblet cells contain an acid mucus and usually aggregate in the apex ('goblet'). All colonic goblet cells would occupy a volume equivalent to that of the exocrine pancreas.

Paneth cells secrete granules rich in lysozyme with marked bacteriolytic properties. Paneth cells may act as stationary phagocytes. They are capable of digesting *Hexamita muris trophozoites* or spiral micro-organisms[19,20] and may thus control the intestinal flora.

There is a normal expression of *HLA-DR-like antigens* by human epithelial cells of the villi in the small intestine and by the epithelium of the colon in chronic inflammatory bowel disease[21,22] (Figure 8). These membrane-bound glycoproteins are probably involved in antigen recognition and initiation of immune responses[23] (Figure 10).

An organ-specific antigen, confined to goblet cells and intestinal glycocalyx[24], could be involved in autoimmune phenomena of certain chronic inflammatory conditions of the gastrointestinal tract. Circulating antibodies specific for antigens on the surface of, or adjacent to, colonic epithelia are present in up to 60% of patients with ulcerative colitis or granulomatous colitis (Crohn's disease)[25].

Epithelium: kinetics

Proliferation and regeneration of epithelial cells take place in the deeper parts of the crypts. The different cell types originate from a pluripotent stem cell of the crypt base.

The normal rate of cell production in the murine small intestine is about 10^8 cells per day[26,27]. The rate of migration of the epithelial sheet over the villous surface ensures complete replacement of the intestinal lining in approximately 2–3 days. Similar estimates have been made in many species. Renewal time in man has been estimated to be 4–6 days[28]. A gradual morphological and functional differentiation occurs during the migration from the crypt base to the surface epithelium. An extrusion zone can be detected at the top of the villi.

Various *exogenous and endogenous regulatory factors* can influence the cell kinetics of the intestinal mucosa (Figure 9). Different *trophic factors* control mucosal growth and atrophy[29]. Pregnancy and lactation, both associated with increased caloric requirement and food intake, result in an

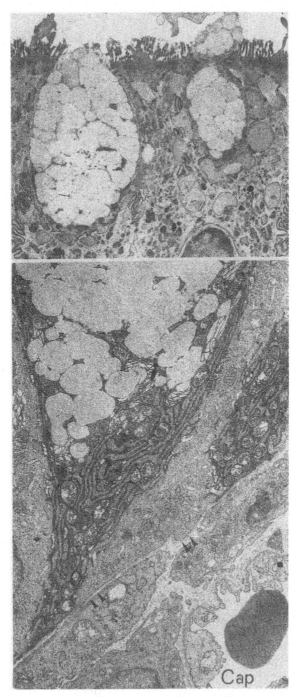

Figure 7 Electron micrographs of human intestinal goblet cells with prominent basal and lateral rough endoplasmic reticulum, extensive Golgi complex and apical mucus granules which are released into the intestinal lumen (top). Epithelial basement membrane (arrow heads), blood capillary (Cap); ×5700

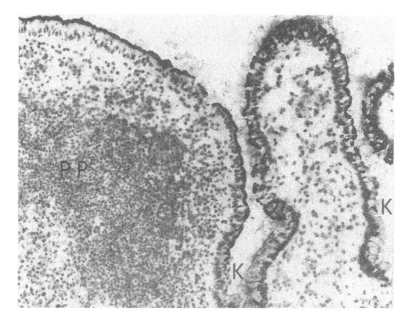

Figure 8 Immunohistochemical demonstration of HLA-DR antigen on the epithelium of the human small intestine, namely on the follicle-associated epithelium of a Peyer's patch (PP) and on the villous epithelium but not on the crypt epithelium (K). Frozen section, alkaline phosphatase antin-alkaline phosphatase method, ×220

increased absorptive area in hamsters: intestinal length, villus height and mucosal area increase. The intestine responds in a similar way to diabetes mellitus, to increased feeding rates (hyperphagia) and to surgical resection of diseased intestinal segments. In contrast, starvation leads to mucosal atrophy and decreased absorption rates. These effects are not abolished by parenteral nourishment. Much of the trophic response of the intestinal mucosa appears to result from direct effects of luminal contents on the enterocytes. Indirect effects are mediated by hormones, e.g. gastrin, glucagon, enteroglucagon, cholecystokinin, secretin, insulin and prolactin, by pancreatic and biliary secretion, and possibly by nerves[29].

The epithelial life cycle is significantly shaped by the *microbial status of the intestine*. There are striking differences between the intestine of germ-free and conventional animals. The wall of the small intestine of germ-free animals of many species is thinner and less well hydrated than in conventional counterparts[30]. The intestinal villi of germ-free animals are more slender and longer than those of conventional animals, the epithelia are more uniform[31], and the total surface area is reduced by about 10 to 30%. In the absence of the bacterial flora, the renewal of the epithelium is markedly retarded[31]. The mitotic index of crypt cells is lower in germ-free than in conventional animals, the generation cycle prolonged, and the pool of proliferating cells smaller. The transit time of epithelial cells moving along

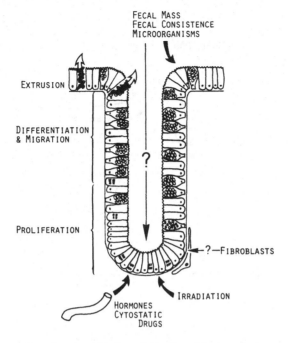

Figure 9 Factors influencing the epithelial cell kinetics of the intestinal mucosa

the villus is also prolonged in germ-free animals. Germ-free animals have fewer lymphocytes, particularly intraepithelial lymphocytes, plasma cells (particularly IgA-cells[32]) in the lamina propria of the gut than conventional animals[31]. The development of Peyer's patches also depends on the microbial status of the host.

The normal flora may reduce several absorptive functions of the gut[33,34].

ANTIGEN UPTAKE

Most potential food antigens are broken down before absorption. The bulk of luminal contents flows through the centre of the gut. Thus, most potential antigens in the gut lumen never reach the mucosa. Absorptive cells may take up small particles by pinocytosis and shuttle them into phagolysosomes, where they are degraded and destroyed resulting in *antigen degradation* (Figure 10). However, a permanent uptake of macromolecules, mostly derived from food and the gut microflora, without degradation takes place. Although this amount of antigens is proportionately small, it is certainly an essential component of the gastrointestinal immune reactivity. The HLA-DR-like antigens expressed by the human gut epithelia (Figure 8) may play a role for the *presentation* of foreign antigens to the local immune system by the epithelia cells[21,23,35,36] (Figure 10).

13

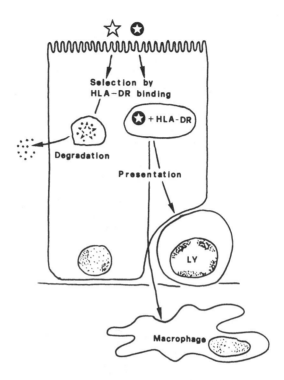

Figure 10 Antigen uptake by enterocytes and the hypothetical role of class II MHC molecules (HLA-DR): the non-selectively absorbed antigenic material is selected by the genetically encoded restricted sequence of the individual's class II molecule (HLA-DR). Those peptides selected for may be presented directly to T cells. Alternatively, the class II molecule may act as a receptor, shuttling immunologically relevant sequences of the antigenic material across the cell in a protected endosome compartment. After release of the antigen at the basolateral cell membrane, the class II 'receptor' then recycles. Non-immunogenic material (that does not bind to class II) would pass on to the lysosome compartment for terminal degradation[23]

The *macromolecules may penetrate* (a) through usual epithelial cells and at particular sites (see below); (b) through intercellular tight junctions because of cellular breakdown – this may occur in malnutrition or under the influence of alcohol; and (c) at the tips of the villi through the major cellular extrusion zones[37-39].

The uptake of intestinal contents has also been studied by use of *particles*. Ingested latex[40] or carbon particles[41] gradually accumulate in the lymphatic follicles of Peyer's patches. Later, these particles appear in draining lymph nodes and lymphoid collections elsewhere in the body. Large molecules and particulate matter travel across the apical epithelium to the basolateral interepithelial space, then across the gaps in the intestinal epithelial basement membrane. The macromolecules may be taken up by local macrophages. They gain access to local lymph nodes or directly to the blood capillaries. The extent to which particulate matter crosses the villous epithelium is not well known. Starch particles[42] and even asbestos[43] may cross the intestinal epithelium, reach the systemic circulation and appear in the urine.

Immunologic contact sites

The main site for the uptake of macromolecules is the epithelium overlying aggregated (Peyer's patches, appendix vermiformis) or solitary lymphatic follicles (Figure 11). The *follicle-associated epithelium* has a sheet of columnar epithelial cells with interspersed membranous (M) epithelial cells[44,45]. The surface membrane of these M cells has no microvilli, but many small projecting folds, microfolds, and small pits (Figures 12 and 13). They contain few if any lysosomes[46]. The M cells attach to regular absorptive cells by tight junctions and form a lattice work with many interstitial intraepithelial lymphocytes. M cells are instrumental for the transepithelial transport of potenially antigenic material, such as horseradish peroxidase[44,47,48] or carbon particles[41] (Figure 13). The M cell is an ideal gateway for the presentation of enteric antigens to the cells of the immune system. A similar mechanism exists in the bronchus-associated lymphatic tissue and in the bursa of the chicken cloaca[49].

Human M cells have been demonstrated in the appendix vermiformis[50] and in Peyer's patches[45]. Many, if not all, M cells probably derive from undifferentiated crypt cells[51].

In experiments with isolated intestinal loops, certain antigens elicit specific secretory antibody only when introduced into loops containing Peyer's patches[52]. The function of solitary lymphatic follicles may be similar to that of Peyer's patches[53]. Hence, Peyer's patches, solitary lymphatic follicles and the vermiform appendix appear to be specialized immunologic contact organs of the gut.

Are M cells channels for infection?

The follicle-associated epithelium, in particular the M cell, is a weak link in the mucosal barrier (Figures 14 and 15). It does not produce the secretory component and therefore lacks the protection of secretory IgA antibodies[35,53a] (Figure 14). The M cells are not common sites of microbial penetration[54]. However, they may endocytize non-invasive *Vibrio cholerae* in the rabbit[55]. M cells provide specific routes of entry for reoviruses from the intestinal tract into the systemic circulation[56,57]. The protozoan, *Giardia lamblia*, penetrates through gaps in the Peyer's patch epithelium[58]. The gaps may be due to rupture of M cells distended by intraepithelial lymphocytes. In Crohn's disease, ulcerations in the vicinity of M cells in Peyer's patches in an otherwise apparently unaffected intestinal epithelium suggest that penetration of an unknown antigen may result in a hyperstimulation of the local immune system and to harmful effects[59,60]. Recently, it has been shown that the adherence of epithelial cells overlying intestinal lymphoid follicles is

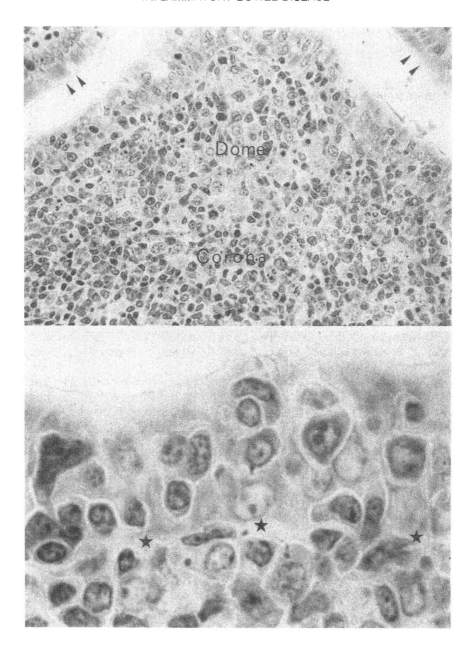

Figure 11 Photomicrographs of the follicle-associated epithelium covering the dome area of a murine Peyer's patch. Top: the nuclei of the follicle-associated epithelium can be seen in various levels, whereas nuclei of the villous epithelium (arrow heads) are typically located at the base of the cells. Dome area with lymphocytes, macrophages and some plasma cells. Bottom: higher magnification showing many intraepithelial lymphocytes. Epithelial basement membrane (asterisks). Semithin sections, toluidine blue. Top: ×520; bottom: ×800

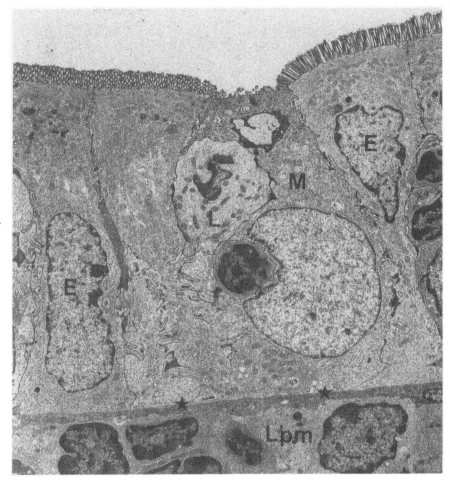

Figure 12 Electron micrograph of an M (membranous) cell (M) with short and irregular microfolds in the follicle-associated epithelium of a murine Peyer's patch. Underneath the M cell are intraepithelial lymphocytes (L) associated with the M cell. E = enterocyte; Lpm = lamina propria mucosa. × 8300

more labile than that of villus and colonic epithelial cells[61]. This fact may be of pathophysiologic significance in ulcerative processes of the follicle-associated epithelium.

Antigen uptake is age dependent

In premature infants, more alimentary antigens appear to be absorbed than in older infants and in adults. In pigs, calves and some small animals (rodents), specific or non-specific, energy-dependent transport systems mediate the uptake of macromolecules by columnar epithelia during the

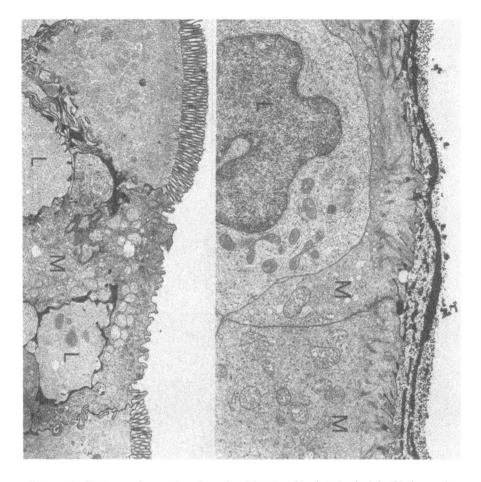

Figure 13 Electron micrographs of murine M cells after intraluminal instillation and sequential uptake of horseradish peroxidase (black reaction products). Top: 10 min after instillation, the reaction products cover the microvilli of the M cells and are seen in intermicrovillous pits. Note the numerous 'empty' cytoplasmic vacuoles of the M cells. Bottom: one hour after instillation, the reaction products are seen in some cytoplasmic vesicles of the M cell (M) and in the epithelial interstices around lymphocytes (L). 3.3'-diaminobenzidine tetrachloride, H_2O_2. Top: ×11 400; bottom: ×8100

postnatal period. Some animals, e.g. pigs, are agammaglobulinaemic at birth and obtain their first antibodies passively through a Fc receptor-associated postnatal uptake. Antigen IgG complexes traverse the gut epithelium of neonatal rats, a capacity formerly attributed only to maternal antibodies[62]. A selective transport of IgG antigen complexes across the intestine may influence the development of systemic immunity and tolerance in the newborn. IgA absorption from colostrum may occur in the newborn infant at least until the third day after birth[63].

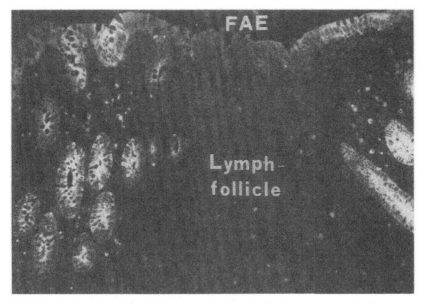

Figure 14 Immunohistochemical demonstration of secretory IgA in the crypt and surface epithelium of the human colon. Note the absence of sIgA in the follicle-associated epithelium (FAE). Indirect immunofluorescence, ×200

The factors which govern '*closure*' of the intestinal transport system are not completely understood. Hormonal factors are involved; cortisone may accelerate the closure[64]. Less bovine serum albumin fed to infant rabbits remains antigenically intact in the serum of breast-fed rabbits than in bottle-fed animals[65]. Newborn infants and guinea pigs fed with cow's milk fomula showed a persistently higher intestinal permeability than the naturally fed groups throughout the first week[66].

Antibodies present in the *breast milk* may limit the uptake of macromolecules and prevent intestinal infection. Breast milk has been shown to protect against neonatal septicaemia[67]. It does not prevent colonization of the intestine by Gram-negative, potentially pathogenic bacteria, but breast milk IgA prevents contact between these micro-organisms and the mucosal membranes[68-71]. Human milk is rich in secretory IgA antibodies against a large number of O, K, H and pilus antigens of enterobacteriaceae[72]. The milk antibodies have arisen in response to microbial antigens in the Peyer's patches, and the patch lymphocytes, mainly switched to IgA production, home also to the mammary glands (see below, Figure 20). As a result, the milk contains large amounts of secretory IgA antibodies against the microbes present in the mother's and the infant's environment. The importance of this is illustrated by the fact that protection in breast-fed infants against infections caused by *V. cholerae, Campylobacter* and enterotoxin-producing *E. coli*, relates to the level of secretory IgA antibodies in the mother's milk against these pathogens[72,73].

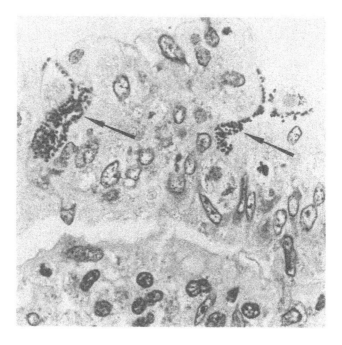

Figure 15 Photomicrograph. Follicle-associated epithelium with bacteria in the human appendix vermiformis. Semithin section, Giemsa, ×750

Observations in lambs show that intact lymphocytes of maternal origin are able to enter the neonatal intestine, especially during the period before closure, and subsequently appear in lymphoid tissue[74]. This suggests another mechanism by which the mother may transfer immunity to the suckled young which would represent a further manifestation of the common mucosal immune system.

Studies on the intestinal uptake of 1.8 μm particles in young (24 days) and aged (18 months) mice indicated that aged mice exhibited significantly more particle accumulation in Peyer's patches than young mice[75].

Secretory IgA and antigen uptake

IgA-class antibodies are secreted by the epithelium and at its surface *reduce antigen absorption*[76-78]. Persons suffering from a selective IgA deficiency absorb more antigens, and hence develop greater immune responses against dietary antigens than normal adults[79]. The mechanisms are poorly understood. Antigen complexed with IgA and trapped at the enterocyte surface might be more susceptible to degradation by pancreatic enzymes[80].

Disease and increased antigen uptake

It has been suggested that a number of diseases may be associated with increased uptake of intestinal antigens, such as coeliac disease, allergic gastroenteropathies, inflammatory bowel disease, viral and bacterial enteritis, parasitic infestations of the intestinal tract, and other diseases that cause changes in the villous architecture (i.e. severe protein-caloric malnutrition, radiation enteritis)[65,78,81,82].

Increased permeability to polyethylene glycol 4000 in rabbits with experimental immune complex-mediated *colitis*[83] supports the hypothesis that inflammation is associated with significant alterations of mucosal permeability and alteration of the mucosal block[60]. This has been demonstrated in ileal segments of patients with *Crohn's disease*, where an increased absorption of polyethylene glycol 600 was demonstrated peroperatively compared with patients with colonic carcinoma[84]. Other studies using different methods confirmed the altered permeability in Crohn's disease, not only in the presence of overt small bowel involvement but also when inflammation is apparently confined to the colon[85,86].

Abnormal intestinal permeability in *coeliac disease* can be demonstrated by the ^{51}Cr-EDTA absorption test, urinary recovery of orally administered isotope being increased in untreated coeliac disease[87]. The observation that treated patients also have a persisting abnormality of permeability to EDTA has prompted the suggestion that an increased intestinal permeability is relevant to the pathogenesis of coeliac disease[88].

Also in *extraintestinal disease*, there have been studies on the possible relevance of abnormalities of intestinal permeability to pathogenesis – notably, in atopic eczema[89] and rheumatoid arthritis[90], in which permeability of high-molecular-weight polymers of polyethylene glycol is abnormal. The altered permeability in rheumatoid arthritis may be an effect of treatment since non-steroidal anti-inflammatory drugs will affect intestinal permeability[91].

A transient increased macromolecular permeability was found in viral enteritis in piglets and in conventional and germ-free mice studying the epithelial transport of horseradish peroxidase[92,93].

Bidirectional transport

The intestinal epithelium is able to excrete substances of high molecular weight into the intestinal lumen (Figure 16). Three routes exist within the villus: between the cells, through the cells, or at the cell extrusion zone[94]. Since both albumin and peroxidase can be taken up at the lateral membrane of the epithelial cell, presumably by pinocytosis, analogous substances of high molecular weight might be excreted via the same route or by extrusion together with epithelial cells. The follicle-associated epithelium thus efficiently transports macromolecules in both directions[95]. Tubular vesicles within the enterocyte mediate the transport of macromolecules[96].

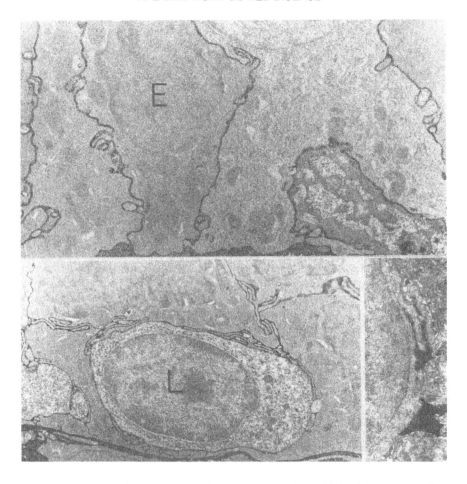

Figure 16 Electron micrographs. Experiment demonstrating the bidirectional transport in murine gut epithelium. Thirty minutes after the intravenous application of horseradish peroxidase, the black reaction products can be seen in the lamina propria and in the epithelial interstices of the jejunum (top) and of the colon (bottom). E = enterocyte; L = intraepithelial lymphocyte; 3.3'-diaminobenzidine tetrachloride, H_2O_2 ×8650. Inset: intraepithelial lymphocyte with reaction products. ×14 250

LYMPHOCYTES IN THE EPITHELIUM: AN IMMUNOLOGICAL COMPARTMENT

Lymphocytes are often found in the interstitial spaces of the epithelium[97] (Figures 16 and 17). They constitute a specialized immunological compartment[98] sharing characteristics with cells found in the epithelium of the respiratory tract and gall bladder[99]. The intestinal epithelium contains as many lymphocytes as does the spleen. These intraepithelial lymphocytes are functionally competent cells, and not merely senescent cells[100], and they differ from the cells in the lamina propria[99]. In mice, the intraepithelial

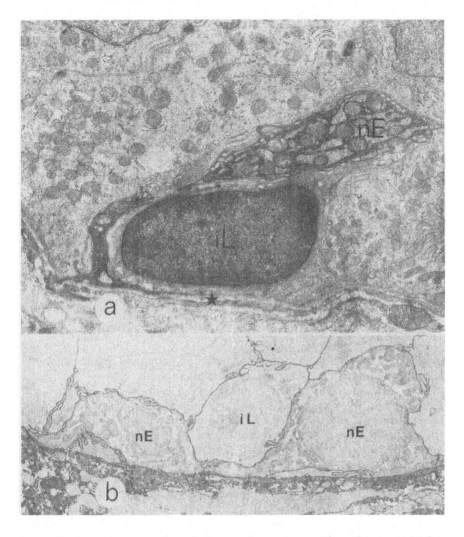

Figure 17 Electron micrographs of the colonic mucosa in ulcerative colitis: intraepithelial lymphocytes (iL) typically situated near the epithelial basement membrane (*) adjacent to necrotic epithelial cells (nE). The interstitial space is 'stained' *in vitro* by horseradish peroxidase (bottom). a: ×11 700; b: ×10 270

lymphocytes are *mainly T cells*[101]. In the human intestinal mucosa, most intraepithelial lymphocytes appear to be T cells of cytotoxic or suppressor immunophenotype (CD8$^+$)[102]. Their secretion products (lymphokines) may have several effects on the epithelium[13]. Intraepithelial lymphocytes and spleen cells, but not bone marrow cells, are able to secrete a factor capable of inducing Ia antigen expression on rat intestinal epithelia *in vitro*[103]. Possibly, the lymphocytes migrate into the crypt epithelium and reach the surface epithelium while being activated (Figure 18). T lymphocytes

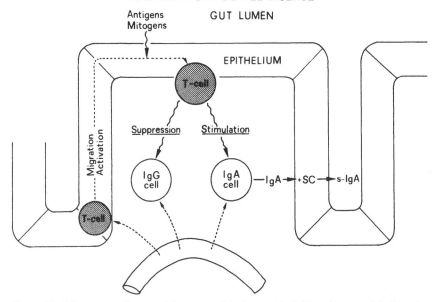

Figure 18 Migratory pathway and functions of the intraepithelial lymphocytes of the intestine (hypothesis)

returning to the lamina propria of the bowel may suppress IgG-production, while they stimulate IgA-synthesis by mucosal plasma cells[77,104,105].

There is a significantly raised number of T cells in the *follicle-associated epithelium* of Peyer's patches and solitary lymphatic follicles compared with the epithelium of distant villi. The T cells tend to be clustered in all layers of the epithelium, being more numerous adjacent to the M cells (Figures 11 and 12). The ratio of $CD4^+$ to $CD8^+$ T cells (about 4:10) was found to be significantly higher in the follicle-associated epithelium than in the villous epithelium (about 0.6:10) of the human small intestine[106]. This suggested that the follicle-associated epithelium may be involved to a greater extent in induction of helper T cell function, perhaps depending on luminal antigens transported by M cells, whereas the villous epithelium may be more involved in stimulation of suppressor T cell functions[106].

Recent investigations of the *T-cell receptors* of the intraepithelial lymphocytes and their relationship to the epithelium have led to new concepts of their function[107,108], although direct demonstration of their physiological role in the immune response has not been elucidated yet[109].

Only 1–2% of T lymphocytes in systemic lymphoid organs or blood, of mice and men, express the γ/δ T-cell receptor (TCR) for antigen; this minor fraction consists mainly of cells that carry the CD3 antigen but not the CD4 or CD8 antigens: hence, they are termed $CD3^+CD4^-CD8^-$ or double negative. It was therefore remarkable when intraepithelial lymphocytes isolated from the murine gut were reported to be exclusively $CD3^+CD4^-CD8^+$ and, by immunoprecipitation, seemed to bear mainly γ/δ TCR[110]. A tissue-specific distribution of TCR subtypes has been proposed, but has received a sceptical response[109,111]. Although 80% of the γ/δ T cells in the

24

human intestinal mucosa were localized in the epithelial layer, these cells represented only 5 to 10% of all CD3[+] T cells in this microenvironment, as most of the human intestinal intraepithelial lymphocytes express the α/β TCR[111,112]. It was concluded from this study that γ/δ T cells represent a sizeable subpopulation of T cells in the human intestine. But this subpopulation may expand in pathological states as in coeliac disease[111,113,114].

The expression of CD8[+] on γ/δ intraepithelial lymphocytes strongly suggests that these cells will be specific for class I MHC molecules, as CD8 expression is associated with class I MHC recognition, and isolated CD8 binds class I MHC molecules. The γ/δ T-cell recognition of autologous class IB MHC molecules, expressed by epithelial cells under conditions of stress, might be an effective, if seemingly primitive, means of epithelial defence. This recognition event should lead to destruction of the stressed epithelial cell[107,108,110] (Figure 17). This form of defence at the immunological frontiers, outside the epithelial basement membranes, could be highly effective. Epithelia that lose a cell or two rapidly cover such lesions by migration of healthy cells into open areas. As long as an infected or a transformed cell is killed before spread across the basement membrane can occur, neither infection nor malignancy can ensue[115]. It is tempting to speculate that this present-day frontier is also the site in which cell-mediated immunity originated, and that this 'new' component of the immune system is actually the oldest.

MUCOSAL LAMINA PROPRIA: A DIFFUSE LYMPHOID ORGAN

The mucosal epithelium is intimately associated with an equally dynamic mesenchymal component, the lamina propria. Stromal cells, fibroblasts in particular, are closely involved in epithelial differentiation during normal development, and in maintaining the differentiated phenotype of epithelial cells in adult tissues[116-118]. Fibroblasts adjacent to the intestinal epithelium accompany the migrating epithelium from the crypt to the villus[119].

The plasma cells, lymphocytes, macrophages, eosinophilic granulocytes, mast cells, the solitary and the aggregated lymphatic follicles constitute a diffuse lymphoid organ that belongs to the intestinal immune system (Table 1).

There are many *T and B lymphocytes* in different states of activation distributed in the lamina propria. The proportion of T cells is larger than that of B cells. Most of the T cells have surface characteristics of helper or inducer cells. The ratio of CD4[+] to CD8[+] is about 2:1, as it is found in the blood and lymph nodes[98,120]. These cells predominantly provide help for IgA and IgM synthesis as it has been found in the human intestinal lamina propria[121,122].

About 90% of the intestinal *plasma cells* normally produce and secrete dimeric IgA (Figure 19). Upon secretion, IgA penetrates into the epithelia where it is bound to the secretory component and extruded as *secretory IgA* (Table 2). The secretory component is synthesized by epithelial cells. It protects the IgA-molecules in the gut against degradation by enzymes and toxins[123,124].

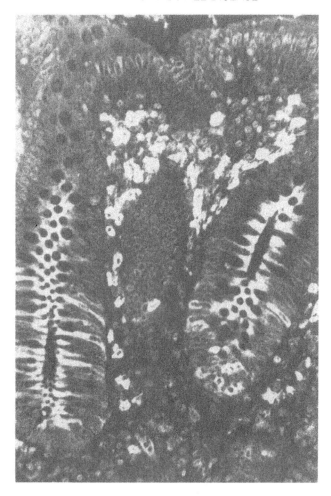

Figure 19 Immunohistochemical demonstration of IgA in the human colonic mucosa in numerous plasma cells of the lamina propria, and in the epithelium. Indirect immunofluorescence; ×330

Table 1 Intestinal immune system in man: cellular and structural elements

Lymphocytes in	{ epithelium lamina propria follicles
Plasma cells Macrophages, mast cells, granulocytes	
Peyer's patches Solitary lymphatic follicles Appendix vermiformis Mesenteric lymph nodes	

Table 2 Secretory IgA: Regulation of Local Immunohomiostasis

Formation of secretory IgA-antigen complexes suppresses:

Bacterial adherence
Bacterial invasion
Viral infections
Antigen uptake
Ig-synthesis of other plasma cell classes
Antigenic stimulation of local lymphocytes
Competitive antigen binding to IgG, IgM;
   therefore complement activation
Competitive antigen binding to IgE;
   therefore hyperimmune reactivity, allergy

Common mucosal immune system

The migrational pathways of enteric immunocytes are intricate. The intestinal IgA-cells are primed in the Peyer's patches, possibly to some extent also in the solitary lymphatic follicles. The maturing cells migrate into the thoracic duct via the mesenteric lymph nodes (Figure 20). Having reached the systemic circulation, they return to the gut mucosa as IgA-secreting plasma cells or their immediate precursors[125,126,141,142]. This journey from the gut-associated lymphoid tissue back to the gut lamina propria

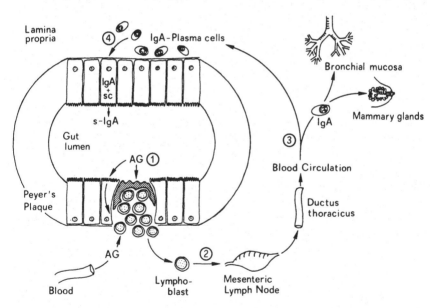

Figure 20 Stimulation and circulation of intestinal IgA precursor cells. **1** Uptake of luminal antigen (AG) through the follicle-associated epithelium of Peyer's patches. **2** Migratory pathway of maturing lymphoblasts through mesenteric lymph node and thoracic duct into the systemic circulation. **3** IgA cells or their immediate precursors home onto the gut mucosa (and to mammary glands or bronchial mucosa) where they secrete IgA in response to antigenic stimulation **4**

27

takes about 4 to 6 days[125]. However, many of the mature IgA-precursor cells may also home in on the connective tissue of other secretory structures, such as mammary glands, salivary glands, bronchial tissue and of the genitourinary tract and constitute 'a common mucosal immune system'[127].

The tissue-specific homing of blood-borne lymphocytes is regulated by interactions with the endothelium of specialized venules in organized lymph nodes and mucosal lymphoid tissues. Recently, a 'vascular addressin' in the

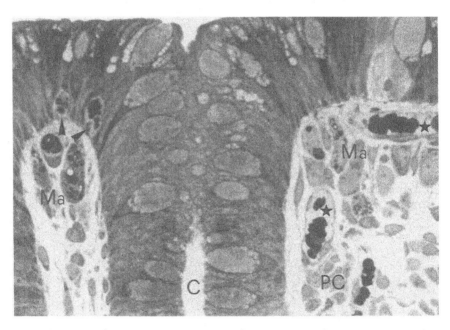

Figure 21 Photomicrograph of the upper parts of the human colonic mucosa. Subepithelial macrophage clusters (Ma), cytoplasmic projections of macrophages into the epithelial interstice (arrow heads), and plasma cell cluster (PC). * = capillary; C = crypt. Semithin section, toluidine blue; ×600

mouse has been identified as a tissue-specific endothelial-adhesion molecule for lymphocytes, and it has been concluded that it could regulate lymphocyte traffic into the mucosal tissues by mediating attachment of blood-borne cells to the endothelium[128].

Macrophages

Clusters of macrophages with morphological signs of increased activity are found under the surface epithelium (Figure 21). There are no macrophages within the epithelial layer. However, cytoplasmic extensions often reach into the epithelial interstices where they contact intraepithelial lymphoctyes. This may express functional interactions.

Ingested carbon particles cross the epithelium of Peyer's patches in mice and appear in subepithelial macrophages[41]. Later, carbon-laden macrophages were present in all areas of Peyer's patches. Approximately eight days elapsed between gavage and appearance of carbon-laden macrophages in germinal centres. Carbon was evident in Peyer's patches and mesenteric lymph nodes four months after cessation of carbon ingestion. The mobility of macrophages was thought to play a role in this distribution. Solitary lymphatic follicles along the intestine handled the carbon in a manner similar to the follicles aggregated in Peyer's patches. Through phagocytosis, interaction with lymphocytes, production of lysozyme and other substances, macrophages contribute to the intestinal mucosal block (Figure 3).

GUT-ASSOCIATED LYMPHOID TISSUE (GALT)

The GALT consists of distinct aggregates of lymphoid cells located in the intestinal mucosa and submucosa, in Peyer's patches, appendix vermiformis, solitary lymphatic follicles, and in the mesenteric lymph nodes. Together with the diffusely scattered mucosal lymphocytes and plasma cells, the GALT forms the intestinal immune system (Table 1).

Peyer's patches occur in the antimesenteric part of the whole mammalian small intestine[129]. They are white, oval to rectangular, slightly raised aggregates of at least five lymphatic follicles of variable size (maximum length: 25 cm)[130]. Peyer's patches are usually larger and more abundant in the ileum but they do occur in the duodenum and jejunum as well.

In humans, the number of patches and follicles *changes with age*. The average number of patches increases from about sixty at 24–29 weeks of gestation to about 240 at the age of 12–14 years, and it decreases to about 100 in persons of more than seventy years of age[130].

Histologically, the nuclei of the flat follicle-associated epithelium are located at various distances from the basement membrane, whereas those of the villous epithelium are located at the base of the cells (Figure 11). The follicle-associated epithelium has few goblet cells, contains specialized M cells and many lymphocytes, mainly T cells (Figures 11–13). The typical lymphatic follicle, situated below the associated epithelium, contains three zones (Figures 11 and 22):

(a) A *dome region* with an associated corona is located immediately beneath the epithelium. The dome contains many large or medium-sized lymphocytes, few small lymphocytes and plasma cells, and many macrophages that contain debris, lipofuscin-like material and, in certain species, bacterial remnants.

(b) The corona surrounds a large *germinal centre* and separates the follicle from the surrounding interfollicular area. The structure of the germinal centre[131] and its proliferative activity[132] resemble that of germinal centres in other lymphoid organs.

(c) The *thymus-dependent area* because it contains mainly small T lymphocytes clustered between large follicles[133].

29

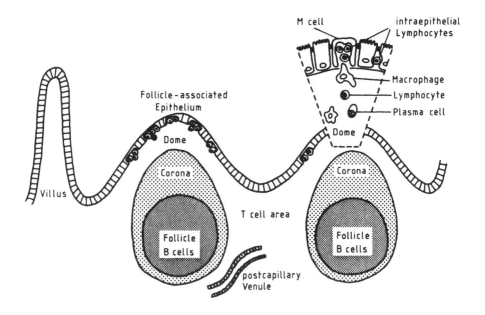

Figure 22   Structure of Peyer's patches (see text)

In addition, there are Ia-positive, interdigitating cells[131]. Many venules with a tall endothelium are present in this region. They correspond to the postcapillary venules in lymph nodes, important sites for the migration of lymphocytes into tissues.

Plasma cells are mainly present in the dome region and within the dome epithelium (Figure 11). Local production of IgG has been demonstrated in Peyer's patches of rats and mice[134-137], and it has been recently shown that there is a remarkably high proportion (38%) of IgG immunocytes among the Ig-producing cells found in the dome area of human Peyer's patches[138]. The significance of this finding is discussed in the chapter on the vermiform appendix.

Solitary lymphatic follicles abound throughout the intestinal tract, particularly in the colon and rectum, with an average of 3–4 follicles per square centimetre in the large intestine[139]. They have a diameter of 0.5–1.0 mm (Figure 23). A germinal centre may be present. The associated epithelium contains M cells[140]. Solitary lymphatic follicles are presumably structural and possibly functional equivalents of Peyer's patches[53,140].

Mesenteric lymph nodes receive the lymph from the small and large intestine in humans. The lymphatics run along the mesenteric arteries. Mesenteric lymph nodes have many lymphoblasts precommitted to IgA synthesis[142].

The *appendix vermiformis* of man is a blind tubular protrusion of the caecum that measures 5–10 mm wide and 2–20 cm long. It has mostly been regarded as a purely vestigial organ. This assumption is based on its small

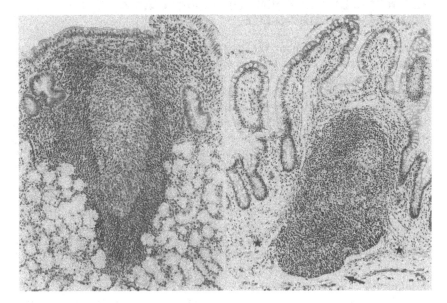

Figure 23 Photomicrographs of solitary lymphatic follicles with germinal centres and lymph sinus (arrow) in the human intestinal mucosa (lamina muscularis mucosae with asterisks). Left: duodenum; right: ileum; ×80

size and lack of digestive function. This is in contrast to the enormous caecum and appendix of the rabbit or of small rodents, where cellulose is broken down into carbohydrates by bacterial action. However, Berry[143] found that the lymphoid tissue of the large intestine tends to aggregate in a specially differentiated part of the caecum, the vermiform appendix, as a species ascends on the scale of vertebrates. In primate *phylogenesis*, the length of the appendix progressively increases as the caecum shrinks in relation to the total colon length. An appendix began to develop in certain Old World monkeys and grew to full size in anthropoid apes; far from being a vestigial organ, its progressive enlargement during primate phylogenesis suggests a functional role[144].

The *structure* of the lymphatic follicles in the human appendix, and of their associated epithelium, is similar to those of Peyer's patches (Figures 11–15). Studies of the rabbit appendix have suggested that it plays a role in the intestinal immune system. Lymphatic follicles are absent at birth[145,146] and they fail to develop after early ligation of the appendix[147]. Elimination of the flora by appendicostomy and sterilization of the lumen causes rapid reduction in size and number of the lymphatic follicles[148].

It seems justified to assume that the function of the lymphatic follicles of the appendix is analogous to that of the Peyer's patches in having the capacity to generate IgA-cell precursors that migrate via lymph and blood to the distant gastrointestinal lamina propria mucosae (Figure 20). There is evidence to suggest that gastrointestinal immunocytes of other isotypes than IgA likewise originate in lymphoepithelial structures[149].

POSTNATAL DEVELOPMENT OF HUMAN GALT AND MAINTENANCE DURING LIFE

There is general agreement that the mass of lymphoid tissue in humans declines as age increases. The spleen undergoes an unexplained increase in weight in middle age before further decline occurs. The number of germinal centres in cervical lymph nodes and the spleen also reduces with age. The human serum antibody response to a variety of bacterial and viral antigens declines in old age[150]. Much of the conflicting information extracted from studies on human subjects must be regarded critically, since the elderly may be regarded as a self-selecting population, or alternatively may be subject to various complications as a consequence of other medical problems or pharmacological treatment.

Although an age-related decline in systemic immunity is documented, little is known about the development of the human GALT after birth and its maintenance during life. Except for some epidemiological data that demonstrate a correlation between increasing age and an increase in the incidence of infectious diseases in the gastrointestinal and respiratory tracts, there is little clinical evidence concerning age-related alterations in mucosal immunity[151].

We have studied the *human appendix vermiformis* to obtain information on (a) the postnatal development of the lymphoid tissue and the time of appearance of plasma cells containing immunoglobulins (Ig); (b) the distribution of the Ig classes in mucosal plasma cells versus age; and (c) the size of the organ and the amount of lymphoid tissue during adult life.

We have examined 190 human appendices without histological signs of active inflammation or luminal obliteration which had been removed 'incidentally' from individuals 1 day to 89 years old.

We measured weight, length and diameter of the specimens and volumes. We counted the lymphatic follicles and germinal centres, measured the mucosal areas and the areas of the lymphatic follicles and germinal centres. Mean values were calculated for each appendix. Serial sections were stained by the peroxidase-anti-peroxidase (PAP) method for IgA, G, M, and E, respectively. For each Ig class, all stained cells were counted in the whole mucosal area of 3 sections taken from the proximal, middle and distal parts.

Median and mean values of the morphometric parameters were almost identical. In the first year after birth, the elongation rate exceeded the increase in volume; length and volume reached maximum values in the first decade and remained constant during adult life; there was no decrease in volume in old age.

The *mucosal area* increased rapidly, reached a maximum during the first year and remained constant thereafter, even in old persons.

There were only very few and small *lymphatic follicles* in the appendix of the newborn (Figure 24). Germinal centres did not appear until the 4th week after birth. Thereafter, the number of both structures increased in parallel and reached a peak in the second decade. After a more rapid decrease in the third decade, these values decreased very slightly after the 5th decade.

There were few *plasma cells* present during the first months after birth (Figure 25). The highest plasma cell numbers were measured in the first

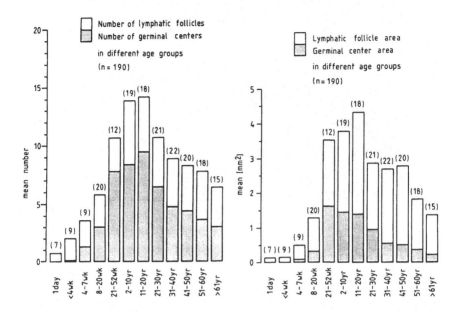

Figure 24 The lymphatic parenchyma of the human appendix vermiformis. Left: the number of lymphatic follicles and germinal centres per cross section (mean values) versus age. Right: the areas of lymphatic follicles and germinal centres per cross section (mean values) versus age

decade. After a decrease in the second decade, their number remained almost constant until old age.

In the appendix of the newborn, we did not observe cells containing immunoglobulins, but the secretory component of IgA was already detectable in the epithelium. The first mature plasma cells appeared 2 weeks after birth. After 4 weeks, there was marked increase in IgA and IgM cells; the number of IgM cells even exceeded that of IgA cells. Twenty weeks after birth, the number of IgA cells reached a maximum value that changed little until old age (Figure 25). Two months after birth, IgM and IgG cell numbers showed an inverse relationship until old age: the IgM cell population decreased while the number of IgG cells increased. The IgE cell number was low (1–2%) in all age groups with a small peak during the first 2 weeks after birth (Figure 25).

In conclusion, for the first 2 weeks after birth, the appendix lacks mature plasma cells and secretory IgA. After that period, there is a rapid rise in the number and a marked predominance of IgM-containing cells, complete by the age of 2–3 months. The rise in IgA-containing cells is much slower. Although large numbers of these cells are found at the age of one month, there is a further increase up to 5 months. Thereafter, the IgA-cell population remains constant until old age.

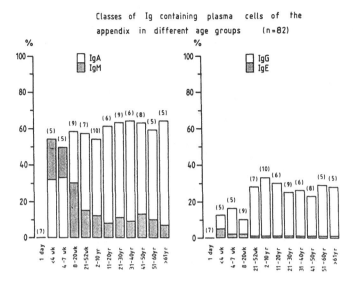

Figure 25 The lymphatic parenchyma of the human appendix vermiformis: distribution of the main immunoglobulin classes of the mucosal plasma cells versus age

Our observations are in accordance with the findings of a study on intestinal specimens and biopsy material from infants 2 hours to 6 months old[152]. In a study on small intestinal mucosa of infants from birth to 21 months of age, the mucosa from parenterally fed children who had received little or no intestinal milk showed significantly fewer immunoglobulin containing cells than those who had been fed normally[153]. Lack of stimulation by food and bacterial antigens may contribute to immunoglobulin containing cells failing to occur in these parenterally fed neonates.

Unexpectedly, anti-*Escherichia coli* IgA and IgM in saliva and meconium have been reported as present already in the first day after birth[154,155]. In one case, these antibodies were found in the newborn of a mother who was deficient in IgA and IgM, indicating foetal production. The stimulus for this foetal production is discussed, and a theory that it may be induced by anti-idiotype antibodies transferred via the placenta, is presented. Anti-idiotype antibodies have been shown to be effective stimulus for protective anti-*E. coli* antibody production in newborn mice[156].

Foreign proteins tend to be absorbed in antigenic form, especially in young infants[157-159]. Absorption of macromolecules was significantly less strong in immunized rats than in controls, suggesting that the absorption of undigested macromolecules is inhibited by local excretion of antibodies[160]. In man, this immune barrier in the intestine is provided by the secretory immunoglobulins, mainly by secretory IgA but also by IgM (see above). Our results show that the human intestine lacks this system during the first two weeks after birth. This deficiency in secretory immunoglobulins is probably the most important factor in the high permeability of the neonatal intestine, which allows formation of antibodies to foreign proteins and may play a part in the pathogenesis of food allergy[161,162].

On the other hand, it is suggested that the intestinal immune system of the newborn is geared towards development of tolerance. Immunologic tolerance to indigenous bacteria and other immunologic factors influencing intestinal flora, have recently been discussed by van der Waaij[163]. This ability of the intestinal immune system to induce oral tolerance seems to decline with age and has been reported in aging mice[164].

The high proportion of IgG plasma cells (30%) in the appendix is also found in Peyer's patches of rats, mice and humans (see above). The high local production of IgG differs markedly from the much lower values observed in the other gut mucosa. This difference can be ascribed to preferential accumulation of IgG immunocytes adjacent to the numerous lymphatic follicles in the appendix. Bjerke et al.[165] presume that this accumulation reflects local terminal maturation of B cells belonging to relatively mature memory clones. Parrot[166] has suggested that some migration of blasts takes place directly from Peyer's patches to nearby crypt regions; these blasts may mainly end up as IgG immunocytes in the follicle-associated mucosal zone. Generation of such clones in lymphoepithelial structures may depend on the magnitude of topical immunological stimulation and apparently increases in the order Peyer's patches, appendix vermiformis, and tonsils[165]. It is assumed that the potency of lymphatic tissue to function as a precursor source of relatively immature B cell clones that can emigrate and seed secretory sites may hence be inversely related to the local IgG response[165].

There appears to be no decrease in size of the normal appendix and only a slight involution of lymphoid tissue with age. Nor does the average number of solitary lymphatic follicles in the intestine of humans obviously decrease in old age[139]. Even in old persons, there are still well-developed lymphoid tissues and many mature plasma cells present. Our findings contrast with the reported involution with age of the lymphatic tissue in other organs. Most experimental studies on gastrointestinal immunity failed to detect an age-related decline in immunoglobulin titres in the gut lumen[167-170]. Thus, structure and presumably function of the GALT differ from those of extraintestinal lymphatic tissue[171,172].

NEUROIMMUNOENDOCRINOLOGY

The immune system and the two other great systems of the body, the nervous and the endocrine system, are functionally connected. Neuroimmunoendocrinology describes the mutual influences of one system upon another, thus indicating the ways by which they communicate[173].

After antigenic challenge, the immune system can synthesize various hormones which appear similar to products of endocrine glands. For instance, immunocytes will produce adrenocorticotropic hormone, ACTH, and endorphins (which are derived from a large precursor protein propiomelanocortin, POMC). Chemically, the leukocyte and the pituitary ACTH appear to have similar sequences. Thyroid stimulating hormone, growth hormone and even chorionic gonadotropic hormone can also be synthesized after appropriate mitogenic and antigenic challenge. All these observations have led to the suggestion that immunocytes can function as endocrine cells.

Furthermore, cells of the immune system show apparently similar control mechanisms to the pituitary gland since, for instance, they will synthesize ACTH in response to corticotrophin releasing factor (CRF). Cells of the immune system are a source of neuroendocrine peptides and the immune system functions as a sensory organ, recognizing stimuli not recognized by the central and the peripheral nervous system.

Various hormone and neuropeptide receptors are found on mononuclear leukocytes indicating that, for the receptors that have been characterized in some detail at the molecular level, such as the VIP receptor and the endorphin receptor, there appears to be a similarity of structures between the nervous cells and the immunocytes.

By means of autonomic noradrenergic sympathetic innervation of the primary and secondary lymphoid organs (thymus, lymph nodes, spleen), immune responses can be modified, perhaps through the presence of adrenoreceptors on lymphocytes.

Various neuropeptides may influence immune functions, such as antibody production, cellular cytotoxicity, T-cell mitogenesis and γ-interferon production. Therefore, the effects of endorphins, enkephalins, arginine-vasopressin, thyroid stimulating hormone (TSH), vasoactive intestinal peptide (VIP), growth hormone, prolactine, somatostatin and substance P have been investigated to some extent. Since an immunocyte can synthesize a neuropeptide (e.g. endorphin or met-enkephalin) for which it possesses a receptor, it is suggested that an immunocyte can function in an autocrine or a paracrine way.

Interleukines, as secretory products mainly of cells of the immune system, such as interferons, IL-2 and IL-1, have hormonal activities. The IL-1 hormonal activity appears to be interesting mainly with regard to the communication pathways existing between the immune system and the other systems. Released after antigenic challenge, IL-1 will act on the hypothalamus or on the hypophysis, stimulating ACTH release which, in turn, by enhanced cortisol production, may shut off the immune response. Tumour necrosis factor and interferons, IL-2 and IL-1, may act on the hypothalamus producing fever.

Since the immune, the nervous and the endocrine system of the intestines reveal particularly close topological associations and vast extensions, the neuroimmunoendocrinological interactions may have a particular significance in the intestinal tract.

ACKNOWLEDGEMENTS

We thank Ms I. Blaha, Ms M. Economou and Ms C. Krähenbühl for excellent technical help.

References

1. Dickman, M.O., Chappelka, A.R. and Schaedler, R.W. (1976). The microbial ecology of the upper small bowel. *Am. J. Gastroenterol.*, **65**, 57-62

2. Hill, M.J. and Drasar, B.S. (1975) The normal colonic bacterial flora. *Gut*, **16**, 318-323
3. Savage, D.C. (1977). Microbial ecology of the gastrointestinal tract. *Ann. Rev. Microbiol.*, **31**, 107-133
4. Cooperstock, M.S. and Zedd, A.J. (1983). Intestinal flora of infants. In Hentges, D.J. (ed.) *Human Intestinal Microflora in Health and Disease.* (Academic Press: New York)
5. Bennet, R. and Nord, C.E. (1989). The intestinal microflora during the first weeks of life: Normal development and changes induced by caesarean section, pre-term birth and antimicrobial treatment. In Grubb, R., Midtvedt, T. and Norin, E. (eds.) *The Regulatory and Protective Role of the Normal Microflora*, pp. 19-34. (New York: Stockton Press)
6. Editorial (1981). Oral encounters with antigen. *Lancet*, **1**, 702
7. Bockman, D.E., Boydston, W.R. and Beezhold, D.H. (1983). The role of epithelial cells in gut-associated immune reactivity. *Ann. N. York Acad. Sci.*, **409**, 129-144
8. Filipe, M.I. (1979). Mucins in the human gastrointestinal epithelium: A review. *Invest, Cell Pathol.*, **2**, 195-216
9. Nimmerfall, F. and Rosenthaler, J. (1980). Significance of the goblet-cell mucin layer, the outermost luminal barrier to passage through the gut wall. *Biochem. Biophys. Res. Commun.*, **94**, 960-966
10. Clamp, J.R. (1980). Gastrointestinal mucus. In Wright, R. (ed.) *Recent Advances in Gastrointestinal Pathology*, pp. 47-58. (London-Philadelphia-Toronto: Saunders)
11. Walker, W.A., Wu, M. and Bloch, K.J. (1977). Stimulation by immune complexes of mucus release from goblet cells of the rat small intestine. *Science*, **197**, 370-371
12. Lake, A.M., Bloch, K.J., Sinclair, K.J. and Walker, W.A. (1980). Anaphylactic release of intestinal goblet cell mucus. *Immunology*, **39**, 1-6
13. Castro, G.A. (1982). Immunological regulation of epithelial function. *Am. J. Physiol.*, **243**, G321-G329
14. Wilson, T.H. (1962). *Intestinal Absorption.* (Philadelphia-London-Toronto: Saunders)
15. Matsudaira, P.T. and Burgess, D.R. (1982). Organization of the cross-filaments in intestinal microvilli. *J. Cell Biol.*, **92**, 657-664
16. Drenckhahn, D. and Gröschel-Steward, U. (1980). Localization of myosin, actin, and tropomyosin in rat intestinal epithelium: Immunohistochemical studies at the light and electron microscopic levels. *J. Cell Biol.*, **86**, 475-482
17. Rodewald, R., Newman, S.B. and Karnovsky, M.J. (1976). Contraction of isolated brush borders from the intestinal epithelium. *J. Cell Biol.*, **70**, 541-554
18. Ito, S. (1965). The enteric surface coat on cat intestinal microvilli. *J. Cell Biol.*, **27**, 475-491
19. Erlandsen, S.L. and Chase, D.G. (1972). Paneth cell function: Phagocytosis and intracellular digestion of intestinal microorganisms. I. *Hexamita muris. J. Ultrastruct. Res.*, **41**, 296-318
20. Erlandsen, S.L. and Chase, D.G. (1972). Paneth cell function: Phagocytosis and intracellular digestion of intestinal microorganisms: II. Spiral microorganisms. *J. Ultrastruct. Res.*, **41**, 319-333
21. Scott, H., Solheim, B.G., Brandtzaeg, P. and Thorsby, E. (1980). HLA-DR-like antigens in the epithelium of the human small intestine. *Scand. J. Immunol.*, **12**, 77-82
22. Chiba, M., Iizuka, M. and Masamune, O. (1988). Ubiquitous expression of HLA-DR antigens on human small intestinal epithelium. *Gastroenterol. Jpn.*, **23**, 109-116
23. Bland, P. (1988). MHC class II expression by the gut epithelium. *Immunol. Today*, **9**, 174-178
24. Roche, J.K., Cook, S.L. and Day, E.D. (1981) Goblet cell glycoprotein: An organ-specific antigen for gut. Isolation, tissue localization and immune response. *Immunology*, **44**, 799-810
25. Gebbers, J-O. (1981).*Colitis ulcerosa: Immun- und Ultrastrukturpathologie.* (Stuttgart-New York: Thieme).
26. Altmann, G.G. and Enesco, M. (1967). Cell number as a measure of distribution and renewal of epithelial cells in the small intestine of growing and adult rats. *Am. J. Anat.*, **121**, 319-324
27. Hagemann, R.F., Sigdestad, C.P. and Lesher, S. (1970). A quantitative description of the intestinal epithelium of the mouse. *Am. J. Anat.*, **129**, 41-49
28. Weinstein, W.M. (1974). Epithelial cell renewal of the small intestinal mucosa. *Med. Clin. N. Am.*, **58**, 1375-1382

29. Diamond, J.M. and Karasov, W.H. (1983). Trophic control of the intestinal mucosa. *Nature (London)*, **304**, 18
30. Thompson, G.R. and Trexler, P.C. (1971). Gastrointestinal structure and function in germ-free or gnotobiotic animals. *Gut*, **12**, 230–239
31. Abrams, G.D., Bauer, H. and Sprinz, H. (1963). Influence of the normal flora on mucosal morphology and cellular renewal in the ileum. A comparison of germ-free and conventional mice. *Lab. Invest.*, **12**, 355–363
32. Crabbé, P.A., Bazin, H., Eyssen, H. and Heremans, J.F. (1968). The normal microbial flora as a major stimulus for proliferation of plasma cells synthesizing IgA in the gut. The germ-free intestinal tract. *Int. Arch. Allergy*, **34**, 362–368
33. Ford, D.J. and Coates, M.E. (1971). Absorption of glucose and vitamins of the B complex by germ-free and conventional chicks. *Proc. Nutr. Soc.*, **30**, 10A
34. Reddy, B.S., Pleasants, J.R. and Wostmann, B.S. (1969). Effects of intestinal microflora on clacium, phosphorus, and magnesium metabolism in rats. *J. Nutr.*, **99**, 353–359
35. Bjerke, K. and Brandtzaeg, P. (1988). Lack of relation between expression of HLA-DR and secretory component (SC) in follicle-associated epithelium of human Peyer's patches. *Clin. Exp. Immunol.*, **71**, 502–507
36. Natali, P.G., DeMartino, C., Quaranta, V., Nicotra, M.R., Frezza, F., Pellegrino, M.A. and Ferrone, S. (1981) Expression of Ia-like antigens in normal human nonlymphoid tissues. *Transplantation*, **31**, 75–78
37. Jackson, D., Walker-Smith, J.A. and Phillips, A.D. (1982) Passive diffusion in small intestinal mucosa in childhood. *Histopathology*, **6**, 689–702
38. Bjarnason, I., Ward, K. and Peters, T. (1984). The leaky gut of alcoholism: possible route of entry for toxic compounds. *Lancet*, **1**, 179–182
39. Talbot, R.W., Foster, J.R., Hermon-Taylor, J. and Grant, D.A.W. (1984). Induced mucosal penetration and transfer to portal blood of luminal horseradish peroxidase after exposure of mucosa of guinea pig small intestine to ethanol and lysolecithin. *Dig. Dis. Sci.*, **29**, 1015–1022
40. LeFevre, M.E., Vanderhoff, J.W., Laissue, J.A. and Joel, D.D. (1978). Accumulation of 2-μm latex particles in mouse Peyer's patches during chronic latex feeding. *Experientia*, **34**, 120–122
41. Joel, D.D., Laissue, J.A. and LeFevre, M.E. (1978). Distribution and fate of ingested carbon particles in mice. *J. Reticuloendothel. Soc.*, **24**, 477–487
42. Volkeimer, G. and Schulz, F.H. (1968). The phenomenon of persorption. *Digestion*, **1**, 213–218
43. Cook, P.M. and Olson, G.F. (1979). Ingested mineral fibers: Elimination in human urine. *Science*, **204**, 195–198
44. Owen, R.L. (1977). Sequential uptake of horseradish peroxidase of lymphoid follicle epithelium of Peyer's patches in the normal unobstructed mouse intestine. *Gastroenterology*, **72**, 440–451
45. Owen, R.L. and Jones, A.L. (1974). Epithelial cell specialization within human Peyer's patches: An ultrastructural study of intestinal lymphoid follicles. *Gastroenterology*, **66**, 189–203
46. Owen, R.L., Apple, R.T. and Bhalla, D.K. (1981). Cytochemical identification and morphometric analysis of lysosomes in M cells and adjacent columnar cells of rat Peyer's patches (abstr.). *Gastroenterology*, **80**, 1246
47. Ducroc, R., Hayman, M., Beaufrere, B., Morgat, J.L. and Desjeux, J.F. (1983). Horseradish peroxidase transport across rabbit jejunum and Peyer's patches in vitro. *Am. J. Physiol.*, **245**, G54–G58
48. Keljo, D.J. and Hamilton, J.R. (1983). Quantitative determination of macromolecular transport rate across intestinal Peyer's patches. *Am. J. Physiol.*, **244**, G637–G644
49. Bienenstock, J. and Johnston, N. (1976). A morphologic study of rabbit bronchial lymphoid aggregates and lymphoepithelium. *Lab. Invest.*, **35**, 343–351
50. Bockman, D.E. and Cooper, M.D. (1975). Early lymphoepithelial relationships in the human appendix. A combined light- and electron-microscopic study. *Gastroenterology*, **68**, 1160–1168
51. Bye, W.A., Allan, C.H. and Trier, J.S. (1984). Structure, distribution, and origin of M cells in Peyer's patches of mouse ileum. *Gastroenterology*, **86**, 789–801
52. Cebra, J.J., Kamat, R., Gearhart, P., Robertson, S.M. and Tseng, J. (1977). The

secretory IgA system of the gut. *Ciba Found. Symp.*, **46** (new series), 5-28
53. Keren, D.F., Holt, P.S., Colins, H.H., Gemski, P. and Formal, S.B. (1978). The role of Peyer's patches in the local immune response of rabbit ileum to live bacteria. *J. Immunol.*, **120**, 1892-1896
53a. Pappo, J. and Owen, R.L., (1988). Absence of secretory component expression by epithelial cells overlying rabbit gut-associated lymphoid tissue. *Gastroenterology*, **95**, 1173-1177
54. Owen, R.L. and Nemanic, P. (1978). Antigen processing structures of the mammalian intestinal tract: A SEM study of lymphoepithelial organs. *Scan. Electron. Microsc.*, **2**, 367-378
55. Owen, R.L., Pierce, N.F., Apple, R.T. and Cray, W.C. (1982). Phagocytosis and transport by M cells of intact *Vibrio cholerae* into rabbit Peyer's patch follicles (abstr.). *J. Cell Biol.*, **95**, 446a
56. Wolf, J.L., Rubin, D.H., Finberg, R., Kauffman, R.S., Sharpe, A.H., Trier, J.S. and Fields, B.N. (1981). Intestinal M cells: A pathway for entry of reovirus into the host. *Science*, **212**, 471-472
57. Wolf, J.L., Kauffman, R.S., Finberg, R., Dambrauskas, R., Fields, B.N. and Trier, J.S. (1983). Determinations of reovirus interaction with the intestinal M cells and absorptive cells of murine intestine. *Gastroenterology*, **85**, 291-300
58. Owen, R.L. (1982). Macrophage function in Peyer's patch epithelium. *Adv. Exp. Med. Biol.*, **149**, 507-513
59. Gebbers, J-O. and Otto, H.F. (1981). Immuno- and ultracytochemical observations in Crohn's disease. In Pena, A.S., Weterman, I.T., Booth, C.C. and Strober, W. (eds.) *Recent Advances in Crohn's Disease*. pp. 136-145. (The Hague, Boston, London: Nijhoff)
60. Gebbers, J-O. and Otto, H.F. (1985). Alterations of the intestinal mucosal block in ulcerative colitis and Crohn's disease – immunological and ultrastructural findings, and considerations of the pathogenesis. *Klin. Pädiat.*, **197**, 341-348
61. Pappo, J., Steger, H.J. and Owen, R.L. (1988). Different adherence of epithelium overlying gut-associated lymphoid tissue. An ultrastructural study. *Lab. Invest.*, **58**, 692-697
62. Abrahamson, D.R., Powers, A. and Rodewald, R. (1979). Intestinal absorption of immune complexes by neonatal rats: A route of antigen transfer from mother to young. *Science*, **206**, 567-569
63. Vukavic, T. (1983). Intestinal absorption of IgA in the newborn. *J. Pediatr. Gastroenterol. Nutr.*, **2**, 248-251
64. Morris, B. and Morris, R. (1976). The effects of corticosterone and cortisone on the uptake of polyvinyl pyrrolidone and the transmission of immunoglobulin G by the small intestine in young rats. *J. Physiol.*, **254**, 389-403
65. Udall, J.N. and Walker, W.A. (1982). The physiologic and pathologic basis for the transport of macromolecules across the intestinal tract. *J. Pediatr. Gastroenterol. Nutr.*, **1**, 295-301
66. Weaver, L.T., Laker M.F., Nelson, R. and Lucas, A. (1987). Milk feeding and changes in intestinal permeability and morphology in the newborn. *J. Pediatr. Gastroenterol. Nutr.*, **6**, 351-358
67. Narayanan, I., Prakash, K., Murthy, N.S. and Guiral, V.V. (1984). Randomised control trial of effect of raw and holder pasteurised human milk and formula supplements on incidence of neonatal infection. *Lancet*, **2**, 1111-1113
68. Gothefors, L., Carlsson, B., Ahlstedt, S., Hanson, L.A. and Winberg, J. (1976). Influence of maternal gut flora and colostral and cord serum antibodies on presence of *Escherichia coli* in faeces of the newborn infant. *Acta Paediatr. Scand.*, **65**, 225-232
69. Hanson, L.A., Ahlstedt, S. and Andersson, B. (1984). The immune response of the mammary gland and its significance for the neonate. *Ann. Allergy*, **53**, 576-582
70. Mata, L.J. and Urrutia, J.J. (1971). Intestinal colonization of breastfed children in a rural area of low socio-economic level. *Ann. N. York Acad. Sci.*, **176**, 93-109.
71. Stevenson, D., Young, C., Kerner, J. and Yeager, A. (1985). Intestinal flora in the second week of life in hospitalized preterm infants fed stored-frozen breast-milk or proprietary formula. *Clin. Pediatr.*, **24**, 338-341
72. Hanson, L.A., Adlerberth, I., Carlsson, B., Dahlgren, U., Hahn-Zoric, M., Jalil, F., Khan, S.R., Larsson, P., Midtvedt, T., Robertson, D., Svanborg-Eden, C. and Wold, A. (1989).

Colonization with enterobacteriaceae and immune response, especially in the neonate. In Grubb, R, Midtvedt, T. and Norin, E. (eds.) *The Regulatory and Protective Role of the Normal Microflora*, pp. 59-69. (New York: Stockton Press)

73. Glass, R.L., Svennerholm, A-M., Stoll, B.J., Khan, M.R., Belayed Hossain, K.M., Huq, M.I. and Holmgren, J. (1983). Protection against cholera in breastfed children by antibodies in breast milk. *N. Engl. J. Med.*, **308**, 1389-1392

74. Sheldrake, R.F. and Husband, A.J. (1985). Intestinal uptake of intact maternal lymphocytes by neonatal rats and lambs. *Res. Vet. Sci.*, **39**, 10-15

75. LeFevre, M.E., Boccio, A.M. and Joel, D.D. (1989). Intestinal uptake of fluorescent microspheres in young and aged mice. *Proc. Soc. Exp. Biol. Med.*, **190**, 23-26

76. Lim, P.L. and Rowley, D. (1982). The effect of antibody on the intestinal absorption of macromolecules and on intestinal permeability in adult mice. *Int. Arch. Allergy Appl. Immun.*, **68**, 41-46

77. Swarbrick, E.T., Stokes, C.R. and Soothill, J.F. (1979). Absorption of antigens after oral immunisation and the simultaneous induction of specific tolerance. *Gut*, **20**, 121-125

78. Walker, W.A. and Isselbacher, K.J. (1974). Uptake and transport of macromolecules by the intestine. Possible role in clinical disorders. *Gastroenterology*, **67**, 531-550

79. Cunningham-Rundles, C., Brandeis, W.E., Good, R.A. and Day, N.K. (1978). Milk precipitins, circulating immune complexes, and IgA deficiency. *Proc. Natl. Acad. Sci. USA*, **75**, 3387-3389

80. Bienenstock, J. and Befus, A.D. (1980). Mucosal immunology. A review. *Immunology*, **41**, 249-270

81. Editorial (1981). Oral encounters with antigen. *Lancet*, **1**, 702

82. Editorial (1985). Intestinal permeability. *Lancet*, **1**, 256-258

83. Seidman, E.G., Hanson, D.G. and Walker, W.A. (1986). Increased permeability to polyethylene glycol 4000 in rabbits with experimental colitis. *Gastroenterology*, **90**, 120-126

84. Olaison, G., Leandersson, P., Sjödahl, R. and Tagesson, C. (1988). Intestinal permeability to polyethyleneglycol 600 in Crohn's disease. Peroperative determination in a defined segment of the small intestine. *Gut*, **29**, 196-199

85. Ukabam, S.O., Clamp, R.J. and Cooper, B.T. (1982). Abnormal small intestinal permeability to sugars in patients with Crohn's disease of the terminal ileum and colon. *Digestion*, **27**, 70-74

86. Bjarnason, I., O'Morain, C., Levi, A.J. and Peters, T.J. (1983). Absorption of [51]chromium labelled ethylene diaminetetraacetate in inflammatory bowel disease. *Gastroenterology*, **85**, 318-322

87. Bjarnason, I., Peters, T.J. and Veall, N.A. (1983). A persistent defect in intestinal permeability in coeliac disease demonstrated by a ^{51}Cr EDTA absorption test. *Lancet*, **1**, 323-325

88. Bjarnason, I., Marsh, M.N., Price, A., Levi, A.J. and Peters, T.J. (1985). Intestinal permeability in patients with coeliac disease and dermatitis herpetiformis. *Gut*, **26**, 1214-1219

89. Jackson, P.G., Lessof, M.H., Baker, R.V.R., Ferrett, J. and Macdonald, D.M. (1981). Intestinal permeability in patients with eczema and food allergy. *Lancet*, **1**, 1285-1286

90. Tagesson, C. and Bengtsson, A. (1983). Intestinal permeability to different-sized polyethylene-glycols in patients with rheumatoid arthritis. *Scand. J. Rheumatol.*, **12**, 124-128

91. Bjarnason, I., Williams, P., Smethurst, P., Peters, T.J. and Levi, A.J. (1986). Effect of non-steroidal anti-inflammatory drugs and prostaglandins on the permeability of the human small intestine. *Gut*, **27**, 1292-1297

92. Keljo, D.J., Butler, D.G. and Hamilton, J.R. (1985). Altered jejunal permeability to macromolecules during viral enteritis in the piglet. *Gastroenterology*, **88**, 998-1004

93. Heyman, M., Corthier, G., Petit, A., Meslin, J-C., Moreau, C. and Desjeux, J-F. (1987). Intestinal absorption of macromolecules during viral enteritis: An experimental study on rotavirus-infected conventional and germ-free mice. *Pediatr. Res.*, **22**, 72-78

94. Dobbins, W.O. (1975). Human intestinal epithelium as a biological membrane. In Trump, B.F. and Arstila, A.U. (eds.) *Pathobiology of Cell Membranes*, pp. 441-442. (New York, San Francisco, London: Academic Press).

95. Bockman, D.E. and Stevens, W. (1977). Gut-associated lymphoid tissue: Bidirectional transport of tracer by specialized eptihelial cells associated with lymphoid follicles. *J.*

Reticuloendothel. Soc., **21**, 245-254
96. Rodewald, R. (1980). Distribution of immunoglobulin G receptors in the small intestine of the young rat. *J. Cell Biol.*, **85**, 18-32
97. Gebbers, J-O. and Otto, H.F. (1973). Das Membranverhalten der interepithelialen Lymphocyten des Darmes. Eine elektronenmikroskopische Untersuchung an Ruthenium-Rot gefärbtem Gewebe. *Virchows Arch. A*, **361**, 175-184
98. Janossy, G., Tidman, N., Selby, W.S., Thomas, J.A., Granger, S., Kung, P.C. and Goldstein, G. (1980). Human T lymphocytes of inducer and suppressor type occupy different microenvironments. *Nature (London)*, **288**, 81-84
99. Ernst, P.B., Befus, A.D. and Bienenstock, J. (1985). Leukocytes in the intestinal epithelium: an unusual immunological compartment. *Immunol. Today*, **6**, 50-55
100. Arnaud-Battandier, F., Bundy, B.M., O'Neill, M., Bienenstock, J. and Nelson, D.L. (1978). Cytotoxic activities of gut mucosal lymphoid cells in guinea pigs. *J. Immunol.*, **121**, 1059-1065
101. Guy-Grand, D., Groscelli, C. and Vassalli, P. (1978). The mouse gut T lymphocyte. A novel type of T cell. Nature, origin, and traffic in mice in normal and graft-versus-host conditions. *J. Exp. Med.*, **148**, 1661-1677
102. Selby, W.S., Janossy, G. and Jewell, D.P. (1981). Immunohistological characterization of intraepithelial lymphocytes of the human gastrointestinal tract. *Gut*, **22**, 169-176
103. Cerf-Benussan, N., Quaroni, A., Kurnick, J.T. and Bhan, A.K. (1984). Intraepithelial lymphocytes modulate Ia expression by intestinal epithelial cells. *J. Immunol.*, **132**, 2244-2252
104. Elson, C.O., Heck, J.A. and Strober, W. (1979). T-cell regulation of murine IgA synthesis. *J. Exp. Med.*, **149**, 632-643
105. Brandtzaeg, P., Sollid, L.M., Thrane, P.S., Kvale, D., Bjerke, K., Scott, H., Kett, K. and Rognum, T.O. (1988). Progress report: Lymphoepithelial interaction in the mucosal immune system. *Gut*, **29**, 1116-1130
106. Bjerke, K., Brandtzaeg, P. and Fausa, O. (1988). T cell distribution is different in follicle-associated epithelium of human Peyer's patches and villous epithelium. *Clin. Exp. Immunol.*, **74**, 270-275
107. Raulet, D.H. (1989). The structure, function, and molecular genetics of the gamma/delta T cell receptor. *Ann. Rev. Immunol.*, **7**, 175-207
108. Raulet, D.H. (1989). Antigens for gamma/delta T cells. *Nature (London)*, **339**, 342-343
109. Bluestone, J.A. and Matis, L.A. (1989). TCR gamma/delta cells – minor redundant T cell subset or specialized immune system compartment? *J. Immunol.*, **142**, 1785-1788
110. Goodman, T. and Lefrancois, L. (1988). Expression of the gamma/delta T-cell receptor on intestinal CD8+ intraepithelial lymphocytes. *Nature (London)*, **333**, 855-857
111. Brandtzaeg, P., Halstensen, T.S., Scott, H., Sollid, L.M. and Valnes, K. (1989). Epithelial homing of gamma/delta T cells? *Nature (London)*, **341**, 113
112. Bucy, R.P., Chen, C.-L.H. and Cooper, M.D. (1989). Tissue localization and CD8 accessory molecule expression of T gamma/delta cells in humans. *J. Immunol.*, **142**, 3045-3049
113. Spencer, J., MacDonald, T.T., Diss, T.C., Walker-Smith, J.A., Ciclitira, P.J. and Isaacson, P.G. (1989). Changes in intraepithelial lymphocyte subpopulations in coeliac disease and enteropathy associated T cell lymphoma (malignant histiocytosis of the intestine). *Gut*, **30**, 339-346
114. Spencer, J., Isaacson, P.G., Diss, T.C. and MacDonald, T.T. (1989). Expression of disulfide-linked and non-disulfide-linked forms of the T cell receptor gamma/delta heterodimer in human intestinal intraepithelial lymphocytes. *Eur. J. Immunol.*, **19**, 1335-1338
115. Janeway, C.A. (1988). Frontiers of the immune system. *Nature (London)*, **333**, 804-806
116. Durnberger, H., Heuberger, B. and Schwartz, P. (1978). Mesenchyme mediated effect of testosterone on embryonic mammary epithelium. *Cancer Res.*, **38**, 4066-4070
117. McLoughlin, C.B. (1961). The importance of mesenchymal factors in the differentiation of the chick epidermis. II. Modification of the epidermal differentiation by contact with different types of mesenchyme. *J. Embryol. Exp. Morphol.*, **9**, 385-409
118. Ozzello, L. (1980). The epithelial stromal function of normal and dysplastic mammary glands. *Cancer*, **25**, 586-600
119. Marsh, M.N. and Trier, J.S. (1974). Morphology and cellular proliferation of subepi-

thelial fibroblasts in adult mouse jejunum. II. Radioautographic studies. *Gastroenterology*, **67**, 636–642

120. Selby, W.S., Janossy, G., Goldstein, G. and Jewell, D.P. (1981). T lymphocyte subsets in human intestinal mucosa: the distribution and relationship to MHC-derived antigens. *Clin. Exp. Immunol.*, **44**, 453–458

121. Kanof, M.E., Strober, W., Fiocchi, C., Zeitz, M. and James, S.P. (1988). CD4 positive Leu-8 negative helper-inducer T cells predominate in the human intestinal lamina propria. *J. Immunol.*, **14**, 3029–3036

122. Smart, C.J., Trejdosiewicz, L.K., Badr-El-Din, S. and Heatley, R.V. (1988). T lymphocytes of the human colonic mucosa: functional and phenotypic analysis. *Clin. Exp. Immunol.*, **73**, 63–69

123. Brandtzaeg, P. (1983). Immunohistochemical characterization of intracellular J-chain and binding site for secretory component (SC) in human immunoglobulin (Ig)-producing cells. *Mol. Immunol.*, **20**, 941–966

124. Brandtzaeg, P. and Prydz, H. (1984). Direct evidence for an integrated function of J chain and secretory component in epithelial transport of immunoglobulins. *Nature (London)*, **311**, 71–73

125. Hall, J. (1979). Lymphocyte recirculation and the gut: The cellular basis of humoral immunity in the intestine. *Blood Cells*, **5**, 479–492

126. Bienenstock, J. and Befus, A.D. (1980). Mucosal immunology. A review. *Immunology*, **41**, 249–270

127. Bienenstock, J., McDermott, M.R., Befus, A.D. and O'Neill, M. (1978). A common mucosal immunologic system involving the bronchus, breast and bowel. In McGhee, J.R., Mestecky, J. and Babb, J.J. (eds.). *Secretory Immunity and Infection*, pp. 53–66. (New York: Plenum Press)

128. Nakache, M., Berg, E.L., Streeter, P.R. and Butcher, E. (1989) The mucosal vascular addressin is a tissue-specific endothelial cell adhesion molecule for circulating lymphocytes. *Nature (London)*, **337**, 179–181

129. Peyer, J.C. (1677). *Exercitatio Anatomico-medica de Glandulis Intestinorum.* (Schaffhausen, Switzerland)

130. Cornes, J.S. (1965). Number, size, and distribution of Peyer's patches in the human small intestine. I. The development of Peyer's patches. *Gut*, **6**, 225–229

131. Sminia, T., Janse, E.M. and Wilders, M.M. (1982). Antigen-trapping cells in Peyer's patches of the rat. *Scand. J. Immunol.*, **16**, 481–485

132. Faulk, P.W., McCormick, J.N., Goodman, J.R., Yoffey, J.M. and Fudenberg, H.H. (1971). Peyer's patches: Morphological studies. *Cell Immunol.*, **1**, 500–520

133. Joel, D.D., Hess, M.W. and Cottier, H. (1972). Magnitude and pattern of thymic lymphocyte migration in neonatal mice. *J. Exp. Med.*, **135**, 907–923

134. Sminia, T. and Plesch, B.E.C. (1982). An immunohistochemical study of cells with surface and cytoplasmic immunoglobulins in situ in Peyer's patches and lamina propria of rat small intestine. *Virchows Arch (Cell Pathol.)*, **40**, 181–189

135. McClelland, D.B.L. (1976). Peyer's patch-associated synthesis of immunoglobulin in germ-free, specific-pathogen-free, and conventional mice. *Scand. J. Immunol.*, **5**, 909–915

136. Crabbé, P.A., Nash, D.R., Bazin, R., Eyssen, H. and Heremans, J.F. (1970). Immunohistochemical observations on lymphoid tissues from conventional and germ-free mice. *Lab. Invest.*, **22**, 448–457

137. Sminia, T., Janse, E.M. and Plesch, B.E.C. (1983). Ontogeny of Peyer's patches of the rat. *Anat. Rec.*, **207**, 309–316

138. Bjerke, K. and Brandtzaeg, P. (1986). Immunoglobulin- and J chain-producing cells associated with lymphoid follicles in the human appendix, colon and ileum, including Peyer's patches. *Clin. Exp. Immunol.*, **64**, 432–441

139. Dukes, C. and Bussey, H.J.R. (1926). The number of lymphoid follicles of the human large intestine. *J. Pathol. Bacteriol.*, **29**, 111–117

140. Rosner, A.J. and Keren, D.F. (1984). Demonstration of M cells in the specialized follicle-associated epithelium overlying isolated lymphoid follicles in the gut. *J. Leukocyte Biol.* **35**, 397–404

141. McDermott, M.R., O'Neill, M.J. and Bienenstock, J. (1980). Selective localization of lymphoblasts prepared from guinea pig intestinal lamina propria. *Cell Immunol.*, **51**, 345–348

142. McWilliams, M., Phillips-Quagliata, J.M. and Lamm, M.E. (1977). Mesenteric lymph node B lymphoblasts which home to the small intestine are precommitted to IgA synthesis. *J. Exp. Med.*, **145**, 866–872

143. Berry, R.J.A. (1900). The true caecal apex, or the vermiform appendix: Its minute and comparative anatomy. *J. Anat. Physiol.*, **35**, 83–98

144. Scott, G.B.D. (1980). The primate caecum and appendix vermiformix: a comparative study. *J. Anat.*, **131**, 549–563

145. Fridenstein, A. and Goncharenko, I. (1965). Morphological evidence of immunological relationships in the lymphoid tissue of rabbit appendix. *Nature (London)*, **206**, 113–115

146. Stramignoni, A. and Mollo, F. (1968). Development of the lymphoid tissue in the rabbit's appendix. A light and electron microscopic study. *Acta Anat.*, **70**, 202–218

147. Stramignoni, A., Mollo, F., Rua, S. and Palestro, G. (1969). Development of the lymphoid tissue in the rabbit appendix isolated from the intestinal tract. *J. Pathol.*, **99**, 265–269

148. Blythman, H.E. and Waksman, B.H. (1973). Effect of irradiation and appendicostomy on appendix structure and responses of appendix cells to mitogens. *J. Immunol.*, **111**, 171–182

149. Brandtzaeg, P. (1985). Research in gastrointestinal immunology: state of the art. *Scand. J. Gastroenterol.*, **20** (Suppl. 114), 137–156

150. Shinozaki, T., Araki, K., Ushijima, H. and Fujii, R. (1987). Antibody response to enteric adenovirus types 40 and 41 in sera from people of different age groups. *J. Clin. Microbiol.*, **25**, 1679–1682

151. Schmucker, D. and Daniels, C. (1985). Aging, gastrointestinal infections and mucosal immunity. *J. Am. Geriatr. Soc.*, **34**, 377–385.

152. Perkkiö, M. and Savilahti, E. (1980). Time of appearance of immunoglobulin-containing cells in the mucosa of the neonatal intestine. *Pediatr. Res.*, **14**, 953–955

153. Knox, W.F. (1986). Restricted feeding and human intestinal plasma cell development. *Arch. Dis. Child.*, **61**, 744–749

154. Mellander, L. (1985). The development of mucosal immunity in relation to natural exposure and vaccination. *Thesis*, University of Götenborg

155. Mellander, L., Carlsson, B. and Hanson, L.A. (1986). Secretory IgA and IgM antibodies to *E. coli* O and Poliovirus type 1 antigens occur in amniotic fluid, meconium and saliva from newborns. A neonatal immune response without antigenic exposure – a result of anti-idiotypic induction? *Clin. Exp. Immunol.*, **63**, 555–561

156. Stein, K. and Sönderström, T. (1984). Neonatal administration of idiotype or anti-idiotype antibodies primes for protection against *Escherichia coli* K13 infection in mice. *J. Exp. Med.*, **160**, 1001–1011

157. Rothberg, R.M. (1969). Immunoglobulin and specific antibody synthesis during the first weeks of life of premature infants. *J. Pediatr.*, **75**, 391–398

158. Leissring, J.C., Anderson, J.W. and Smith, D.W. (1962). Uptake of antibodies by the intestine of the newborn infant. *Am. J. Dis. Child.*, **103**, 160–168

159. Lippard, V.W., Schloss, O.M. and Johnson, P.A. (1936). Immune reactions induced in infants by intestinal absorption of incompletely digested cow's milk protein. *Am. J. Child.*, **51**, 562–569

160. Walker, W.A., Wu, M., Isselbacher, K.J. and Bloch, K.J. (1975). Intestinal uptake of macromolecules. III. Studies on the mechanism by which immunization interferes with antigen uptake. *J. Immunol.*, **115**, 854–859

161. Matthew, D.J., Taylor, B., Norman, A.P., Turner, M.W. and Soothill, J.F. (1977). Prevention of eczema. *Lancet*, **1**, 321–322

162. Taylor, B., Norman, A.P., Orgel, H.A., Stokes, C.R., Turner, M.W. and Soothill, J.F. (1973). Transient IgA deficiency and pathogenesis of infant atopy. *Lancet*, **2**, 111–113

163. van der Waaij, D. (1988). Evidence of immunoregulation of the composition of intestinal microflora and its practical consequences. *Eur. J. Microbiol. Infect. Dis.*, **7**, 103–106

164. Hosokawa, T., Motoi, S., Aoike, A., Koyama, K., Rokutan, K., Nishi, Y. and Kawai, K. (1988). Effect of aging on immunological memory in gastrointestinal tract induced by sheep red blood cells in mice. *Gastroentrol. Jpn.*, **23**, 13–17

165. Bjerke, K., Brandtzag, P. and Rognum, T.O. (1986). Distribution of immunoglobulin producing cells is different in normal human appendix and colon mucosa. *Gut*, **27**, 667–674

166. Parrott, D.M.V. (1976). The gut-associated lymphoid tissues and gastrointestinal immunity. In Ferguson, A. and MacSween, R.N.M. (eds.) *Immunological Aspects of the Liver and Gastrointestinal Tract*, pp. 1–32 (Lancaster: MTP)

167. Kawanishi, H. and Kiely, J. (1985). Effect of aging on murine gut-associated lymphoid tissue. *Gastroenterology*, **88**, 1440 (abstr.)

168. Senda, S., Cheng, E. and Kawanishi, H. (1986). Aging-associated changes in murine intestinal immunoglobulin secretes. *Gastroenterology*, **90**, 1626–1631

169. Ebersole, J., Smith D. and Taubman, M. (1985). Secretory immune responses in aging rats. I. Immunoglobulin levels. *Immunology*, **56**, 345–351

170. Lim, T., Messiha, N. and Watson, R. (1981). Immune components of the intestinal mucosa of aging and protein deficient mice. *Immunology*, **43**, 401–408

171. Szewczuk, M.R., Campbell, R.J. and Jung, L.K. (1981). Lack of age-associated immune dysfunction in mucosal-associated lymph nodes. *J. Immunol.*, **126**, 2200–2204

172. Hess, M.W., Zimmermann, A., Brun, del Re, G. and Cottier, H. (1975). Immunologische Aspekte gastrointestinaler Neoplasien. *Schweiz. Med. Wochenschr.*, **105**, 570–575

173. Blalock, J.E. and Bost, K.L. (eds.) (1988). *Neuroimmunoendocrinology. Progress in Allergy*, Vol. 43. (Basel: Karger)

2
Genetics of inflammatory bowel disease

A.S. PEÑA

INTRODUCTION

Inflammatory bowel disease (IBD), that is ulcerative colitis and Crohn's disease, may have a common genetic susceptibility and environmental factors may determine the development of one or the other. On the other hand, IBD may be heterogeneous or multifactorial. Heterogeneity is suggested by numerical taxonomy[1], the existence of different clinical patterns with regard to expression and prognosis[2], and the constitution and extent of the histological lesion. Another criterion which seems to suggest heterogeneity is the association with other diseases. Crohn's disease is associated more often with eczema than ulcerative colitis is, and the latter is more often associated with coeliac disease and other autoimmune diseases[3]. In this chapter, the following facets are reviewed: the factors supporting a genetic predisposition, the possible genetic markers for disease susceptibility, and some of the environmental factors which may contribute to the expression of inflammatory bowel disease.

FACTORS SUPPORTING A GENETIC PREDISPOSITION

Familial aggregations

It has long been known that the familial occurrence of ulcerative colitis (UC) and Crohn's disease is increased in patients with IBD[4]. A general prevalence of 7.9% of familial occurrences was found in an unselected population in a well-defined area over a long period of time (Stockholm County, Sweden)[5]. Recently, age-corrected empiric risk estimates for inflammatory bowel disease in the Ashkenazi Jewish population in the United States have been developed[6]. This study demonstrates that there is an increased risk for the offspring, siblings and parents of patients with ulcerative colitis and Crohn's disease. 19.8% of patients with ulcerative colitis had a positive family history. In the study of Stockholm County[5], patients with a positive family history of ulcerative colitis were also found to have a lower age at onset of the disease; this was not the case in the study from Los Angeles[6].

The prevalence of affected first-degree relatives of patients with IBD is higher than expected, and affected uncles, cousins, and grandparents have been reported. For example, in ulcerative colitis, first-degree relatives were found to have a prevalence 15 times higher than non-relatives and the prevalence of Crohn's disease in first-degree relatives was 3.5 times higher than in non-relatives[5].

The segregation of the disease in first-degree relatives supports a multifactorial form of inheritance for Crohn's disease[7] and for ulcerative colitis[5].

Concordant and discordant monozygous twins

The recent report from Sweden[8] on the largest study done so far and the only one based on an unselected twin register, has clearly shown that the genetic contribution is unequivocally stronger in Crohn's disease than in ulcerative colitis. Only one pair among monozygotic twins (6.3%) were concordant for ulcerative colitis and none of the 17 dizygotic pairs were. One the other hand, 8 out of 18 pairs of monozygotic twins (44.4%) were concordant for Crohn's disease compared with only one out of 26 pairs of dizygotic twins. This finding suggests that evaluation based on earlier twin reports with ulcerative colitis, where a higher degree of concordance had been observed, probably overestimated the importance of genetic factors in this disease.

Spouses

Very few cases of ulcerative colitis in husband and wife have been reported. In some of the couples, one of the partners was affected with Crohn's disease instead of ulcerative colitis[9-15] (Table 1). If shared familial environmental agents were the only factors necessary for the expression of the disease, many more cases should exist. However, in Crohn's disease, the situation may be different. The number of spouses reported with Crohn's disease is reaching a value which is probably higher than that expected by chance alone[16-25] (Table 2).

Incidence in different ethnic groups and migrants

Several studies have shown that Jews have a higher incidence than the other races living in the same area. This was first shown in Baltimore[26] in 1960–1963 where Jews had an annual incidence of 13 per 10^5 compared with non-

Table 1 Ulcerative colitis in husband and wife

Authors	Year	Diagnosis	Sex	Country	Age at diagnosis	Site of disease	Family history
Kirsner[9]	1973	UC CD	F M	— —	38 40		Son: UC
Rosenberg et al.[10]	1976	UC CD	F M	USA USA	44 —	Colon Ileum	Son: UC
Craxi et al.[11]	1979	UC UC	F F	Italy			—
Mayberry et al.[12]	1980	CD UC	? ?	UK UK	? ?		
Kirsner[13] (Goodman)	1982	UC CD	M F	USA USA			—
Almy and Sherlock[14]	1966	UC UC	M F	USA USA	— —	Colon Colon	
Bennett et al.[15]	1988	19 IBD couples		USA	?	?	Yes

Table 2 Crohn's disease in husband and wife

Authors	Year	Diagnosis	Sex	Country	Age at diagnosis	Site of disease	Family history
Zetzel[16]	1978 (1963)	CD CD	F M	USA USA	25 37	Terminal ileum / Terminal ileum	Daughter: colon
Whorwell et al.[17]	1978	CD CD	M F	UK UK	49 54	Ileum / Iluem	
Korelitz[18]	1979	CD CD	M F	USA USA			
Whorwell et al.[19]	1981	CD CD	M F	UK UK	26 20	Colon / Ileum	
Rhodes et al.[20]	1985	CD CD CD CD	M F M F	UK UK UK UK	30 28 20 42	Colon, perianal / Ileum, caecum / Ileum, colon / Colon	
Holmes and Paine[21]	1986	CD CD	M F	UK UK	29 32		
Purrman et al.[22]	1987	CD CD	M F	Germany Germany	20 32	Ileum+colon+rectum / Ileum+right colon	(Aunt)
Murray and Thomson[23]	1988	CD CD	M F	Canada Canada	29 25	Ileum+rectum / Ileum+rectum	(Aunt)
Lobo et al.[24]	1988	CD CD	F M	UK UK	?62 ?59	Colon / Colon	
Darchis et al.[25]	1989	CD CD	M F	France France	42 51	Ileum+right colon / Ileum	3 sons: CD 1 daughter

Jewish whites (3.8) and blacks (1.4). Similar figures have been observed in the Cape Town area of South Africa[27] where Jews had an incidence of 17, whites 5, coloureds 1.4 and blacks 0.6 per 10^5 for ulcerative colitis. In the Negev in southern Israel, 58% of the population are immigrants. It has recently been reported[28] that Jews of European and American origin have a significantly higher incidence of ulcerative colitis (10.8 per 10^5) than Jews born in North Africa and the Middle East (5.1 per 10^5) or in Israel (4.1 per 10^5). This study suggests that environmental influences play an important role in the development of inflammatory bowel disease. In the Netherlands, there has been a significant migration of people of Indonesian, Turkish, Moroccan and Surinamese origin into areas such as Leiden[29]. The migration is recent (25–30 years) and the epidemiology of chronic diseases in these groups is not yet clear. In the Leiden area, six cases with proctocolitis amongst the 7037 migrants were identified, compared with none of Crohn's disease. The prevalence of ulcerative colitis in migrants was $85.3/10^5$ (range 35–195, 95% confidence limits) and this was not significantly different from the indigenous Dutch population. In relation to Crohn's disease, 11 patients among Jamaicans living in the UK have been reported[30]. As pointed out by the investigators, the long period spent in the UK by two patients born in Jamaica and the permanent residence of the other nine cases is consistent with the role of environmental factors in the aetiology of the disease and indicates that West Indians are not genetically protected against the development of Crohn's disease.

In summary, the studies performed in families of patients with inflammatory bowel disease and in different ethnic groups indicate that genetic factors play a role in the aetiology of these diseases. Genetic factors seem to be necessary but are not sufficient to develop the disease. It is also clear that real differences exist between ulcerative colitis and Crohn's disease concerning hereditary factors.

ADDITIONAL FACTORS SUPPORTING A GENETIC PREDISPOSITION

Inflammatory bowl disease associated with other diseases

Ankylosing spondylitis

Both ulcerative colitis and Crohn's disease have been found to be associated with ankylosing spondylitis (AS)[31] and the association between ankylosing spondylitis and HLA-B27 is well established[32]. However, the carriage rate of the genetic marker HLA-B27 in IBD patients is lower than in patients with AS alone, although, in some series of patients with UC and spondylitis, as many as 80% had the HLA-B27 antigen.

Psoriasis

Psoriasis coexisting with IBD has also been described. For example, a study from Scotland[33] in 116 patients with Crohn's disease and 88 with ulcerative colitis found that the prevalence of psoriasis was 11.2% and 5.7%, respectively; a prevalence which is significantly higher than in the age- and sex-matched control group, which was 1.5%. One family with cases of psoriasis, psoriatic spondylitis, Crohn's disease, and AS without the HLA-B27 marker has been reported[34].

A relationship between psoriasis, ankylosing spondylitis, sacroiliitis, peripheral arthropathy, and IBD may be explained by common genetic factors. The carriage of HLA-B27 is not necessarily the only marker for predisposition and other factors within the HLA region or in other chromosomes may be relevant to explain the common association.

Atopy and eczema

Atopy and eczema, both of which have a marked hereditary component, have also been reported to be associated with IBD, although not all of the studies have found this association. In a recent international co-operative study[35] performed in 14 centres in nine countries, eczema occurred more frequently in patients with Crohn's disease and their first-degree relatives than in the controls and their families. A similar trend was observed for UC but did not reach statistical significance.

Coeliac disease

With respect to coeliac disease, there have been several case reports of an association with inflammatory bowel disease and, in a recent survey, the siblings of 120 patients with coeliac disease had a twenty-fold higher risk of developing coeliac disease and a fifteen-fold higher risk of developing ulcerative colitis than the controls[36].

Multiple sclerosis

A concurrence of multiple sclerosis and inflammatory bowel disease in families and in patients has been recognized[37-39]. One or more loci contributing specifically to IBD may also determine the susceptibility for multiple sclerosis. On the other hand, a common defect in immune regulation may exist in both diseases, the presence of antilymphocyte antibodies in the serum of patients and their relatives may be a marker for this defect.

Autoimmune disease

Ulcerative colitis has been repeatedly reported in association with several autoimmune diseases, such as autoimmune haemolytic anaemia[40]. Another case where an anti-erythrocyte antibody was present without a haemolysis has been described[41].

Systemic lupus erythematosus and Hashimoto's disease may coexist with ulcerative colitis[42]. More recently, a patient with Crohn's disease and SLE has been reported[43].

Primary sclerosing cholangitis

Primary sclerosing cholangitis (PSC), characterized by an obliterative inflammation and fibrosis of the entire biliary duct system, has been described in association with inflammatory bowel disease. In the vast majority of these patients, IBD preceded PSC and a relationship with severity of inflammatory bowel disease was indicated[44]. A familial coincidence of PSC and ulcerative colitis has been reported[45,46], indicating that certain patients with IBD may be predisposed to suffer from PSC and are at greater risk of developing the disease when the HLA-B8,DR3 is present or other still unknown factors are introduced.

Turner syndrome

Turner syndrome, characterized by phenotypic features, short stature and gonadal dysgenesis, sometimes with horse shoe kidneys, has been associated with Crohn's disease and ulcerative colitis[47]. The association of inflammatory bowel disease with Turner syndrome may be due to hypogonadism according to Turnbull *et al.*[48] since other conditions, like Kallman's syndrome (hypogonadotropic hypogonadism with anosmia), have been found to be associated with ulcerative colitis.

Turcot's syndrome

A case has been reported of Turcot's syndrome, i.e. a hereditary condition of brain tumour and colonic polyps, in a patient who developed adenocarcinoma of the colon and had a daughter with Crohn's disease and a son with duodenal ulcer[49].

Glycogen storage disease type Ib

Glycogen storage disease type Ib (GSD-Ib) is a metabolic disorder characterized by abnormal transport of glucose-6-phosphate into the endoplasmic reticulum. The patients have neutropenia, neutrophil dysfunction and recurrent oral mucosal lesions. Roe *et al.*[50] have observed two boys with GSD-Ib and chronic IBD indistinguishable from Crohn's disease and suggested that the neutrophil abnormality in these patients may be involved in the pathogenesis of IBD. This is particularly interesting in view of the variable deficiencies of neutrophil oxidative metabolism in Crohn's disease[51].

Sarcoidosis

Sarcoidosis and Crohn's disease have been observed in the same family. The father of a family in Finland developed extrathoracic sarcoidosis. Six years later, within the same year, three of his children were examined for sarcoidosis, hypercalciuria, and Crohn's disease affecting the ileum and ascending colon, respectively[52]. The nature of the triggering agent, the primary site of invasion, or additional genetic factors may determine whether sarcoidosis or Crohn's disease will develop.

POSSIBLE MARKERS FOR SUSCEPTIBILITY

Histocompatibility antigens (HLA)

A recent analysis of the available data on HLA-A and -B antigen distributions in patients with Crohn's disease and ulcerative colitis according to mathematical techniques used to aggregate sets of data of different sizes showed that Caucasian individuals with HLA-A2 have a relative risk of 1.25 of developing Crohn's disease, and HLA-B27 and -Bw35 individuals a relative risk of 1.81 and 1.41, respectively, of suffering from ulcerative colitis, whereas, for the latter disease, the relative risk for Japanese with HLA-B5 is 2.79[53].

A recent study from Germany[54] has shown a special type of genetic heterogeneity of patients with ankylosing spondylitis and Crohn's disease. The phenotype HLA-B27,B44 was found to be markedly increased when both diseases coincide. Individuals with this phenotype have a relative risk of 68.8 for the concurrent manifestation of Crohn's disease and ankylosing spondylitis.

Genetic factors play an important predisposing role in the expression of SLE. The association between SLE and DR2 is also of interest in view of the association described between the haplotype A10-B18-DR2 in association with IBD and deficiency of the second component of complement[55] as well as the increased frequency of an allele of C2 and SLE patients[56,57].

Immunoglobulin allotypes

In spite of an earlier report suggesting an association of immunoglobulin allotypes[58], the available evidence seems to indicate that these genetic markers do not play an important role in the susceptibility of individuals to Crohn's disease[59] or ulcerative colitis[60,61].

Complement allotypes

The gene loci coding for the complement components, Bf, C3, and C4, are known to be closely linked to the HLA complex. Slade *et al.* reported for the first time a hereditary complement deficiency, namely C2 deficiency associated with IBD and the A10-B18 HLA haplotype[55]. Danish investigators have studied the polymorphism of complement C3 in IBD. C3 has two common alleles, namely C3F and C3S, which give rise to the phenotypes, F, FS and S. The frequency of the CRF allele was significantly increased in patients with Crohn's disease of the small bowel compared with that in healthy volunteers. The frequency of C3F in ulcerative colitis did not differ from that in controls[62]. More recently, a German group found that, among the complement markers tested, the frequency of the Bf-F allotype was significantly higher in patients with Crohn's disease than in the controls, 65.6% versus 28.3% respectively[63].

Lymphocytotoxic antibodies

Lymphocytotoxic antibodies (LCA) have been found in patients with inflammatory bowel disease and in their healthy relatives[64,65]. These antibodies, which do not detect a genetically determined structural antigen, may be markers for an environmental antigen. LCA in family members were more frequent in consanguineous relatives without close household contact than in control families[64]. These findings suggest that a genetic component may be operative in the expression of the antibody response to an environmental agent. Thus, the available evidence suggests that LCA in IBD might be a manifestation of an immunological abnormality rather than simply markers of viral agents.

Susceptibility factors determining the bacterial flora

International studies have confirmed the finding that patients with Crohn's disease have an abnormal anaerobic flora. Van de Merwe[66] suggested that the genetic predisposition for Crohn's disease is in fact shown by the presence of an abnormal faecal flora in these patients. Identical twins have identical intestinal flora. This hypothesis is interesting because evidence is accumulating that genetic factors control bacterial attachment to the epithelium.

Increased intestinal permeability

Normally the intestine can selectively prevent the absorption of molecules larger than 0.4 nm in diameter and soluble in water.

Hollander et al.[67] of the University of California have found that the intestinal permeability to polyethyleneglycol 400 is increased more than two-fold in patients with Crohn's disease and some of their healthy relatives. These authors have put forward the hypothesis that increased intestinal permeability may be a genetically expressed defect which predisposes individuals to the development of Crohn's disease.

Abnormal permeability of the intestine using different probes has been reported in coeliac disease and in other non-intestinal diseases. However, the interesting association between coeliac disease and ulcerative colitis mentioned above does suggest that careful consideration should be given to these findings. Permeability may be abnormal as a secondary result of inflammation. Lactulose absorption is increased in patients with Crohn's disease. But lactulose, rhamnose, or mannitol failed to detect permeability abnormalities in healthy relatives of patients with Crohn's disease[68].

Colonic glycoproteins

The mucus layer covering the mucosal surface has been analysed with different techniques. Mucin proteins, which are large glycoproteins, are the most important constituents of the mucus layer. Analysis by chromatography in DEAE-cellulose of mucosal scrapings showed six mucin glycoproteins. Podolsky and Isselbacher[69] called these molecules mucin species I, II, III, IV, V, and VI. These investigations have shown that purified colonic mucin from patients with ulcerative colitis has a selective reduction of mucin species IV. Although the significance of this finding is still unknown, recent work suggests that this defect may represent a hereditary defect and therefore a primary abnormality. Järnerot and Podolsky have recently found that identical twins with ulcerative colitis have the same defect (unpublished observations). If this is confirmed, this finding suggests a structural marker involved in the predisposition to develop ulcerative colitis. The defect on its own is not sufficient to acquire the disease since healthy twins also had this defect.

ENVIRONMENTAL FACTORS

The role of dietary practices, water supply, agrarian and urban areas, and other social activities is yet to be clearly defined.

Smoking

There are many studies showing that the relative risk of ulcerative colitis developing in non-smokers is higher compared with smokers[70,71]. Ex-smokers usually develop their disease after stopping smoking[72,73]. Epidemiological studies consistently support the different association of cigarette smoking with ulcerative colitis and Crohn's disease. It has been suggested that in genetically predisposed individuals, the smoking exposure may determine the type of inflammatory bowel disease that will develop[73]. The study of identical twins in Sweden showed that the smoking pattern was similar in concordant and discordant twins. After diagnosis, two healthy monozygotic twins had given up smoking for a mean period of 6.5 years without developing ulcerative colitis. This implies that the sharing of identical genes and smoking patterns is not enough[8]. Other environmental factors should be looked for.

Contraceptive pill

The risk of developing inflammatory bowel disease in oral contraceptive users is definitely increased for Crohn's disease but not for ulcerative colitis[74].

In summary, the environmental factors so far identified, such as dietary factors, smoking patterns, and the use of the oral contraceptive pill, appear to be more important as risk factors for developing Crohn's disease than for ulcerative colitis.

COLORECTAL CANCER RISK

Although population studies such as the study in central Israel[75], have shown a lower risk for malignancy in patients with inflammatory bowel disease, than studies from referral centres, there is a significantly increased risk for adenocarcinoma in these patients. Recently, Gyde et al.[76] have reported in a cohort study from three different centres that patients with ulcerative colitis have an increased risk for colorectal cancer which appears at around the age of 40 years, regardless of the duration and extent of the colitis. They postulate a genetic predisposition for developing colorectal cancer. Delpré et al.[77], on the other hand, have concluded that colorectal cancer in patients with Crohn's disease, whether it represents a genetic predisposition or an acquired condition, continues to be an area of controversy.

Acknowlegements

The author wishes to thank Mrs Maritza Koster-de Vreese and Mrs Nelia Koek-van Beelan for typing the manuscript.

References

1. Hywell Jones, J., Lennard Jones, J.E., Morson, B.C., Chapman, M., Sackin, M.J., Sneath, P.H.A., Spicer, C.C. and Card, W.I. (1973). Numerical taxonomy and discriminant analysis applied to non-specific colitis. Q. J. Med., 169, 715-732
2. Sachar, D.B., Wolfson, D.M., Greenstein, J.A., Goldberg, J., Styczunski, R. and Janowitz, H.D. (1983). Risk factors for postoperative recurrence of Crohn's disease. Gastroenterology, 85, 917-921
3. Peña, A.S., Weterman, I. and Lamers, C.B.H.W. (1987). Predisposing markers and regulating genes in inflammatory bowel disease. In Järnerot, G. (ed.) Inflammatory Bowel Disease, pp. 9-19. (New York: Raven Press)
4. Lewkonia, R.M. and McConnell, R.B. (1976). Familial inflammatory bowel disease: heredity or environment? Gut, 17, 235-241
5. Monsén, U., Broström O., Nordenvall, B., Sörstad, J. and Hellers, G. (1987). Prevalence of inflammatory bowel disease among relatives of patients with ulcerative colitis. Scand. J. Gastroenterol., 22, 214-218
6. Roth, M.P., Petersen, G.M., McElree, C., Vadheim, C.M., Panish, J.F. and Rotter, J.I. (1989). Familial empiric risk estimates of inflammatory bowel disease in Ashkenazi Jews. Gastroenterology, 96, 1016-1020
7. Begleiter, M.L. and Harris, D.J. (1985). Familial incidence of Crohn's disease. Gastroenterology, 88, 221
8. Tysk, C., Lindberg, E., Järnerot, G. and Flodérus-Myrhed, B. (1988). Ulcerative colitis and Crohn's disease in an unselected population of monozygotic and dizygotic twins. A study of heritability and the influence of smoking. Gut, 29, 990-996
9. Kirsner, J.B. (1973). Genetic aspects of inflammatory bowel disease. Clin. Gastroenterol., 2, 557-575

10. Rosenberg, J.L., Draft, S.C. and Kirsner, J.B. (1976). Inflammatory bowel disease in all three members of one family. *Gastroenterology*, **70**, 759–760
11. Craxi, A., Oliva, L. and Di Stefano, G. (1979). Ulcerative colitis in a married couple. *Ital. J. Gastroenterol.*, **11**, 184–186
12. Mayberry, J.F., Rhodes, J. and Newcombe, R.G. (1980). A short report: Familial prevalence of inflammatory bowel disease in relatives of patients with Crohn's disease. *Br. Med. J.*, **280**, 84
13. Kirsner, J.B. (1982). Later development of inflammatory bowel disease in the healthy spouse of a patient. *N. Engl. J. Med.*, **307**, 1148
14. Almy, T.P. and Sherlock, P. (1966). Genetic aspects of ulcerative colitis and regional enteritis. *Gastroenterology*, **51**, 757–761
15. Bennett, R., Rubin, P.H. and Present, D.H. (1988). Inflammatory bowel disease (IBD) in husbands and wives. Frequency of IBD in 35 offspring of 19 couples. *Gastroenterology*, **94**, A611
16. Zetzel, L. (1978). Crohn's disease in a husband and wife, *Lancet*, **2**, 583
17. Whorwell, P.J., Eade, O.E., Hossenbocus, A. and Bamforth, J. (1978). Crohn's disease in a husband and wife. *Lancet*, **2**, 186–187
18. Korelitz, B.I. (1979). From Crohn to Crohn's disease: 1979 an epidemiologic study in New York City. *Mt. Sinai Med. (NY)*, **6**, 433–440
19. Whorwell, P.J., Hodges, J.R., Bamforth, J. and Wright, R. (1981). Crohn's disease in husband and wife. *Lancet*, **1**, 334
20. Rhodes, J.M., Marshall, T., Hamer, J.D. and Allan, R.N. (1985). Crohn's disease in two married couples. *Gut*, **26**, 1086–1087
21. Holmes, G.K.T. and Painter, N.S. (1986). Crohn's disease in married couples. *Gut*, **27**, 350
22. Purrmann, J., Cleveland S., Miller, B. and Strohmeyer, G. (1987). Crohn's disease in a married couple. *Hepato-gastroenterology*, **34**, 132–133
23. Murray, C.J.W. and Thomson, A.B.R. (1988). Marital idiopathic inflammatory bowel disease. *J. Clin. Gastroenterol.*, **10**, 95–97
24. Lobo, A.J., Foster, P.N., Sobala, G.M. and Axon, A.T.R. (1988). Crohn's disease in married couples. *Lancet*, **1**, 704–705
25. Darchis, I., Colombel, J.F., Cortot, A., Devred, M. and Paris, J.C. (1989). Crohn's disease in a married couple and their four children. *Lancet*, **1**, 737
26. Monk, M., Mendeloff, A.I., Seigel, C.I. and Lilienfeld, A. (1969). An epidemiological study of ulcerative colitis and regional enteritis among adults in Baltimore. II. Social and demographic factors. *Gastroenterology*, **56**, 847–857
27. Wright, J.P., Frogatti, J., O'Keefe, E.A., Ackerman, S., Watermeyer, S., Louw, J., Adams, G., Girwood, A.H., Burns, D.G. and Marks, I.N. (1986). The epidemiology of inflammatory bowel disease in Cape Town 1980–1984. *S. Afr. Med. J.*, **70**, 10–15
28. Odes, H.S., Fraser, D. and Kraiec, J. (1986). Inflammatory bowel disease in migrant and native Jewish populations of southern Israel. *Dig. Dis. Sci.*, **31** Suppl. 835, 322
29. Shivananda, S., Peña, A.S., Mayberry, J.F., Ruitenberg, E.J. and Hoedemaeker, Ph.J. (1987). Epidemiology of proctocolitis in the region of Leiden, The Netherlands. *Scand. J. Gastroenterol.*, **22**, 993–1002
30. Fellows, I.W., Mayberry, J.F. and Holmes, G.K.T. (1988). Crohn's disease in West Indians. *Am. J. Gastroenterol.*, **83**, 372–375
31. Davis, P. (1979). Quantitative sacroiliac scintigraphy in ankylosing spondylitis and Crohn's disease: a single family study. *Ann. Rheum. Dis.*, **38**, 241–243
32. Woodrow, J.C. and Eastwood, C.J. (1978). HLA-B27 and the genetics of ankylosing spondylitis. *Ann. Rheum. Dis.*, **37**, 504–509
33. Hickling, P., Bird-Steward, J.A., Young, J.D. and Wright, V. (1983). Crohn's spondylitis: a family study. *Ann. Rheum. Dis.*, **42**, 106–107
34. Yates, V.M., Watkinson, G. and Kelman, A. (1982). Further evidence for an association between psoriasis, Crohn's disease and ulcerative colitis. *Br. J. Dermatol.*, **106**, 323–330
35. Gilat, T., Hacohen, D., Lilos, P. and Langman, M.J.S. (1987). Childhood factors in ulcerative colitis and Crohn's disease. An international cooperative study. *Scand. J. Gastroenterol.*, **22**, 1009–1024
36. Mayberry, J.F., Smart, H.L. and Toghill, P.J. (1986). Familial association between coeliac disease and ulcerative colitis. *J. R. Soc. Med.*, **79**, 204–205
37. Rang, E.H., Brooke, B.N. and Hermon-Taylor, J. (1982). Association of ulcerative colitis

and multiple sclerosis. *Lancet*, **1**, 555
38. Minuk, G.J. and Lewkonia, R.M. (1986). Possible familial association of multiple sclerosis and inflammatory bowel disease. *N. Engl. J. Med.*, **314**, 586
39. Sadovnik, A.D., Paty, D.W. and Yannakoulis, G. (1989). Concurrence of multiple sclerosis and inflammatory bowel disease. *N. Engl. J. Med.*, **321**, 762–763
40. Basista, M.H. and Roe, D.C. (1986). A case presentation of hemolytic anemia in ulcerative colitis and review of the literature. *Am. J. Gastroenterol.*, **81**, 990–992
41. Chiba, M., Nakajima, K., Arakawa, H., Masamune, O. and Narisawa, T. (1988). Anti-erythrocyte antibodies in ulcerative colitis: case report and discussion on the pathophysiology of anti-erythrocyte antibodies. *Gastroenterol. Jpn.*, **23**, 564–569
42. Alarcón-Segovia, D., Herskovic, T., Dearing, W.H., Bartholonew, L.G., Cain, J.C. and Shorter, R.G. (1965). Lupus erythematosus cell phenomenon in patients with chronic ulcerative colitis. *Gut*, **6**, 39–43
43. Nagata, N., Ogawa, Y., Hisano, S. and Veda, K. (1989). Crohn's disease in systemic lupus erythematosus: a case report. *Eur. J. Pediatr.*, **148**, 525–526
44. Stockbrügger, R.W., Olsson, R., Jaup, B. and Jensen, J. (1988). Forty-six patients with primary sclerosing cholangitis: Radiological bile duct changes in relationship to clinical course and concomitant inflammatory bowel disease. *Hepato-gastroenerology*, **35**, 289–294
45. Quigley, E.M.M., LaRusso, N.F., Ludwig, J., MacSween, R.N.M., Birnie, G.G. and Watkinson, G. (1983). Familial occurrence of primary sclerosing cholangitis and ulcerative colitis. *Gastroenterology*, **85**, 1160–1165
46. Silber, G.H., Finegold, M.J., Wagner, M.L. and Klish, W.J. (1987). Sclerosing cholangitis and ulcerative colitis in a mother and her son. Case report. *J. Pediatr. Gastroenterol. Nutr.*, **6**, 6, 147–152
47. Knudtzou, J. and Svane, S. (1988). Turner's syndrome associated with chronic inflammatory bowel disease. A case report and review of the literature. *Acta Med. Scand.*, **223**, 375–378
48. Turnbull, A.J., Law, A. and Peters, T.T. (1988). Ulcerative colitis associated with Kallmann's syndrome. *J. R. Soc Med.*, **81**, 354–355
49. Scapa, E., Umlas, J., Loewenstein, M.S. and Zamcheck, N. (1983). Non familial Turcot's syndrome associated with Crohn's disease and duodenal ulcer in one kindred. *Am. J. Gastroenterol.*, **78**, 411–413
50. Roe, T.F., Thomas, D.W., Gilsanz, V., Isaacs, H. and Atkinson, J.B. (1986). Inflammatory bowel disease in glycogen storage disease type Ib. *J. Pediatr.*, **109**, 55–59
51. Verspaget, H.W., Mieremet-Ooms, M.A.C., Weterman, I.T. and Peña A.S. (1981). Partial defect of neutrophil oxidative metabolism in Crohn's disease. *Gut*, **25**, 849–853
52. Grönhagen-Riska, C., Fyhrquist, F., Hurtling, L. and Koskimies, S. (1983). Familial occurrence of sarcoidosis and Crohn's disease. *Lancet*, **1**, 1287–1288
53. Biemond, I., Burnham, W.R., D'Amaro, J. and Langman, M.J.S. (1986). HLA-A and -B antigens in inflammatory bowel disease. *Gut*, **27**, 934–941
54. Purrmann, J., Zeidler, H., Bertrams, J., Juli, E., Cleveland, S., Berges, W., Gemsa, R., Specker, C. and Reis, H.E. (1988). HLA antigens in ankylosing spondylitis associated with Crohn's disease. Increased frequency of the HLA phenotype B27, B44. *J. Rheumatol.*, **15**, 1658–1661
55. Slade, J.D., Luskin, A.T., Gewurz, H., Kraft, S.C., Kirsner, J.B. and Zeitz, H.J. (1978). Inherited deficiency of second component of complement and HLA haplotype A10, B18 associated with inflammatory bowel disease. *Ann. Intern. Med.*, **88**, 796–798
56. Fu, S.M., Stern, R., Kunkel, H.G., Dupont, B., Hansen, J.A., Day, N.K., Good, R.A., Jersild, C. and Fotino, M. (1975). Mixed lymphocyte culture determinants and C2 deficiency: LD-7a associated with C2 deficiency in four families. *J. Exp. Med.*, **142**, 495–506
57. Glass, D., Raum, D., Gibson, D., Stillman, J.S. and Schur, P.H. (1976). Inherited deficiency of the second component of complement. *J. Clin. Invest.*, **58**, 853–861
58. Kagnoff, M.F., Brown, R.J. and Schanfield, M.S. (1983). Association between Crohn's disease and immunoglobulin heavy chain (Gm) allotypes. *Gastroenterology*, **85**, 1044–1047
59. Biemond, I., de Lange, G., Weterman, I.T. and Peña, A.S. (1987). Immunoglobulin allotypes in Crohn's disease in The Netherlands. *Gut*, **28**, 610–612
60. Gudjonsson, H., Schanfield, M.S., Albertini, R.J., McAuliffe, T.L., Beeken, W.L. and

Krawitt, E.L. (1988). Association and linkage studies of immunoglobulin heavy chain allotypes in inflammatory bowel disease. *Tiss. Antigens*, **31**, 243–249

61. Field, L.L., Boyd, N., Bowen, T.L., Kelly, J.K. and Sutherland, L.R. (1989). Genetic markers and inflammatory bowel disease: Immunoglobulin allotypes (GM,KM) and protease inhibitor. *Am. J. Gastroenterol.*, **84**, 753–755

62. Elmgreen, J., Sørensen, H. and Berkowicz, A. (1984). Polymorphism of complement C3 in chronic inflammatory bowel disease. *Acta Med. Scand.*, **215**, 375–378

63. Kluge, F., Grosse-Wilde, H., Kreeb, G., Doxiadis, I., Vögeler, U., Hoppe-Seyler, P. and Koch, H. (1982). Association between the HLA-linked complement allotype marker Bf-F and Crohn's disease. *Scand. J. Gastroenterol.*, 17 Suppl., **78**, 513

64. Korsmeyer, S.J., Williams, R.C. Jr., Wilson, I.D. and Strickland, R.G. (1976). Lymphocytotoxic and RNA antibodies in inflammatory bowel disease: a comparative study in patients and their families. *Ann. NY Acad. Sci.*, **278**, 574–585

65. Kuiper, I., Weterman, I.T., Biemond, I., Castelli, R., Rood, J.J.V. and Peña, A.S. (1981). Lymphocytotoxic antibodies in patients with Crohn's disease and family members. In Peña, A.S., Weterman, I.T., Booth, C.C. and Strober, W. (Eds.) *Recent Advances in Crohn's disease.* pp. 208–211. (The Hague: Martinus Nijhoff)

66. Van de Merwe, J. (1984). The human faecal flora and Crohn's disease. *Antonie van Leeuwenhoek*, **50**, 691–700

67. Hollander, D., Vadheim, C.M., Brettholz, E., Petersen, G.M., Delahunty, T.J. and Rotter, J.I. (1986). Increased intestinal permeability in patients with Crohn's disease and their relatives. A possible etiological factor. *Ann. Intern. Med.*, **105**, 883–885

68. Katz, K.D., Hollander, D., Vadheim, C.M., McElrey, C., Delahunty, J., Dadufalza, V.D., Krugliak, P. and Rotter, J.I. (1989). Intestinal permeability in patients with Crohn's disease and their healthy relatives. *Gastroenterology*, **97**, 927–931

69. Podolsky, D.K. and Isselbacher, K.J. (1983). Composition of human colonic mucin: selective alternation in inflammatory bowel disease. *J. Clin. Invest.*, **72**, 142–153

70. Smith, M.B., Lashner, B.A. and Hauauer, S.B. (1988). Smoking and inflammatory bowel disease in families. *Am. J. Gastroenterol.*, **83**, 407–409

71. Katschinski, B., Logan, R.F.A., Edmond, M. and Langman, M.J.S. (1988). Smoking and sugar intake are separate but interactive risk factors in Crohn's disease. *Gut*, **29**, 1202–1206

72. Boyko, E.J., Perera, D.R., Koepsell, T.D., Keane, E.M. and Inui, T.S. (1988). Effects of cigarette smoking on the clinical course of ulcerative colitis. *Scand. J. Gastroenterol.*, **23**, 1147–1152

73. Tobin, M.V., Logan, R.F.A., Langman, M.J.S., McConnell, R.B. and Gilmore, I.T. (1987). Cigarette smoking and inflammatory bowel disease. *Gastroenterology*, **93**, 316–321

74. Calkins, B.M., Mendeloff, A.D. and Garland C. (1986). Inflammatory bowel disease in oral contraceptive users. (Letter) *Gastroenterology*, **91**, 523–524

75. Gilat, T., Fireman, Z., Grossman, A., Hacohen, D., Kadish, U., Ron, E., Rozen, P. and Lilos, P. (1988). Colorectal cancer in patients with ulcerative colitis. A population study in central Israel. *Gastroenterology*, **94**, 870–877

76. Gyde, S.N., Prior, P., Allan, R.N., Stevens, A., Jewell, D.P., Truelove, S.C., Lofberg, R., Brostrom, O. and Hellers, G. (1988). Colorectal cancer in ulcerative colitis: a cohort study of primary referrals from three centres. *Gut*, **29**, 206–217

77. Delpré, G., Kadish, V. and Wolloch, Y. (1989). Colorectal cancer and colonic disease: A matter for analysis and reflection. *Gastroenterol. Clin. Biol.*, **13**, 45–50

3
Special aspects of inflammatory bowel disease in children

B.S. KIRSCHNER

The inflammatory bowel diseases, chronic non-specific ulcerative colitis and Crohn's disease, have been increasingly recognized as important clinical entities in paediatric patients. In the following discussion, an overview of selected features of these disorders as they affect children is presented, recognizing that areas relating to genetics, endoscopic and radiological diagnosis, and management (medical, dietary and surgical) are addressed elsewhere in the Symposium.

Epidemiology

An observed change in the frequency of these disorders occurred between the 1950s and the 1980s, during which time Crohn's disease increased while ulcerative colitis stabilized. Recently, Barton et al. reported that the incidence of Crohn's disease in Scottish children increased three-fold between 1968 and 1983, while ulcerative colitis remained unchanged[1]. Farmer and Michener noted that ulcerative colitis was diagnosed twice as often as Crohn's disease in the 1950s but that the reverse is now observed[2]. Children with ulcerative colitis are more likely to have the onset of their disease before 10 years of age (12.8%) than are children with Crohn's disease (5.6%)[3].

Aetiopathogenesis

Although the aetiology of these disorders is unknown, current investigations support the importance of family history[4,5], ethnicity[4] and altered immunological response within the intestine[6-9]. An international multicentre study which compared 499 children and adolescents with IBD with 978 normal controls was unable to discern differences between the two groups with regard to the frequency of breast feeding, formula intolerance in infancy, acute gastrointestinal infection, or parental divorce or death[5].

Of special interest is the work by Mayer et al. who observed that intestinal epithelial cells of patients with IBD stimulated the proliferation of lamina propria lymphocytes to mitogen in contrast to a suppressor effect with normal epithelial cells[6,7]. In addition, recent evidence suggests that HLA-DR markers on colonic epithelial cells may become more readily expressed in patients with Crohn's disease, which may influence their local immune response[9].

CLINICAL DIVERSITY

Intestinal involvement

While we tend to think of Crohn's disease as a single disease entity, the clinical diversity within the patient population is great. The broad range of clinical presentations reflects, in part, the location and extent of disease, severity of the inflammatory response and individual susceptibility to progression or quiescence, as well as extraintestinal manifestations. The majority of children (80%) have ileocolonic involvement, but 10% have either isolated small bowel or colonic disease. The reasons why certain sites are involved in specific patients are unknown, although it is known that family patterns are common with regard to a predominance of CD or UC within multiple relatives of an individual family[4].

Examples of the variety of initial gastrointestinal signs and symptoms of Crohn's disease include: recurrent vomiting (especially with gastroduodenal disease); abdominal pain which is often postprandial with small bowel involvement or related to defecation when the colon is involved; an inflammatory mass (resulting from enteric fistulae); bloody diarrhoea (frequently related to colonic disease); and perianal disease (skin tags, fissures, fistulae and abscesses). The latter complications are relatively common, occurring in 49% of paediatric patients, and are associated with a greater frequency of granuloma formation than is observed in patients without perianal disease[10].

Children with chronic non-specific ulcerative colitis usually have pancolitis (62%), although disease localized to the rectum occurs in 15% of patients[11]. Mir-Madhjessi *et al.* have reported a greater likelihood for proximal extension in paediatric than adult patients[12]. Varying degrees of bloody diarrhoea and abdominal cramping in association with defecation are the predominant symptoms.

Extraintestinal manifestations

The initial presentation of Crohn's disease can be particularly subtle, occurring in the absence of diarrhoea and haematochezia. Intestinal signs and symptoms are often overshadowed by extraintestinal manifestations. Fever is noted in 40% of children at the time of diagnosis, although it may go unrecognized in many cases.

In a series of 58 children with CD, the correct diagnosis was made by the admitting house officers in only 22% of cases[13]. Rheumatological or collagen–vascular diseases were initially considered more likely. This is not surprising since arthritis is observed in 9% of children with UC and 15% with CD[14]. Arthralgias are even more common. Both symptoms usually affect large joints, reflect underlying bowel activity, and resolve within 2–4 weeks with control of the intestinal disease.

Other systemic complications of IBD include mucocutaneous lesions, such as oral ulcers (UC 2%, CD 9%), erythema nodosum (UC 4%, CD 8–15%) and pyoderma gangrenosum (UC 5%, CD 1.3%)[15]. Renal manifestations are calculi (6%), enterovesicular fistulae, hydroureter and hydronephrosis secondary to compression by an inflammatory mass, and, rarely, secondary amyloidosis[16]. Serious cerebrovascular complications manifest by seizures, focal motor disorders, coma and abnormalities in speech have been described in children with UC and CD[17,18]. Both venous thrombosis and cerebral arteritis have been reported. While factors related to a hypercoagulable state (thrombocytosis and reduced antithrombin III) are altered in some patients, no consistent finding is present in all patients.

Growth failure

Impaired linear growth, defined as a fall in height percentile, has been observed in approximately 36% of children with CD and 14% of children with UC at the time of diagnosis[19]. However, growth failure appears to be more frequent when defined as reduced growth velocity in centimeters/year (cm/y) over that expected for normal children of similar age and sex. In a retrospective study, Kanof et al. noted that growth velocity was attenuated in 88% of prepubertal children with CD diagnosed between 1961 and 1985[20]. A review of 25 children with CD, pubertal stages I-II, diagnosed in our institution since 1980 revealed subnormal growth velocity in 60% of patients. This difference may reflect earlier recognition of CD.

Potential mechanisms of growth impairment

Intestinal absorption

In investigating the causes of growth failure in this population, we and others have shown that malabsorption is not a consistent finding. D-xylose absorption, 72-hour fat excretion, and Schilling tests for vitamin B12 are abnormal in only a minority of these children[21-23]. In a small number of patients, Motil et al. reported that mineral losses for zinc, magnesium, calcium and phosphorus exceeded control values[24].

Protein status

We have observed that dietary protein intake exceeds the recommended dietary allowance in our population of children with IBD and growth failure[23]. Motil et al. reported that protein metabolism, as measured by leucine flux, was not significantly different in six patients from sibling controls[25]. Despite these findings, enhanced enteric protein loss, associated with hypoalbuminaemia, occurs in most children during active disease.

Caloric insufficiency

Dietary assessment of growth-impaired children with IBD has consistently documented caloric insufficiency[21-23,26]. The calorie intake does not meet the recommended dietary allowance for age and sex in most instances. It is our impression that this reflects early satiety (particularly with gastroduodenal involvement), and provides some control over the postprandial pain of small bowel disease and increased stool frequency of either small intestinal or colonic involvement.

We have observed that caloric insufficiency is profound in this population. In our series, calorie intake averaged only 54% of the recommended dietary allowance (RDA) for age and sex[23]. Other groups have reported intakes under 80% of recommended[22,26]. Reversal of this undernutrition, whether by enteral or parenteral means, is followed by enhanced growth velocity and, in some instances, achievement of the pre-illness height[25-29].

Limited data are available concerning measurements of energy expenditure in this patient population. Kelts et al. reported that the basal metabolic rate was not increased in 5 growth-impaired children[22]. We measured resting energy expenditure, using the stable isotopes $^2H_2O-H_2^{18}O$, in 6 hospitalized paediatric patients with Crohn's disease and also found that it was not greater than expected[30]. Studies on ambulatory patients, comparing intake and expenditure, are needed to understand this problem more fully.

Endocrine studies

Although secondary growth hormone (GH) deficiency was originally postulated to be the cause of growth failure in these children, subsequent reports by several groups have documented normal GH responses to provocative testing[31-33]. Recently, Farthing et al. noted that spontaneous nocturnal GH secretion may be reduced in some growth-impaired patients and that this correlated with disease activity[33]. Delay in sexual maturation and skeletal maturation frequently accompanies impaired linear growth. Farthing et al. observed that nocturnal gonadotropin concentrations correlated closely with GH secretion and suggested that both aspects of hypothalamic–pituitary function are likely to be affected by disease activity and calorie deprivation[33].

This may explain, in part, along with the change in nutritional status, the reduced somatomedin-C (insulin-like growth factor I) levels that we observed in growth-impaired children in comparison with normally-growing children with IBD[34]. Somatomedin-C levels were measured because of the well-documented effect of fasting and refeeding on somatomedin activity in rats[35]. Somatomedin-C levels in our growth-impaired patients rose three-fold within 4 weeks of medical nutritional therapeutic intervention. We found a strong correlation with calorie intake (r = 0.68) and growth velocity (r = 0.71) but not with serum albumin concentration (r = 0.32)[34].

Thyroid function studies are usually normal except for transiently reduced tri-iodothyronine in malnourished patients[36]. The diurnal variation in cortisol secretion, despite the discomfort of bowel disease, is maintained[36].

Reversal of growth failure

The importance of nutrition support in reversing growth failure was suggested by Layden *et al.* following their use of total parenteral nutrition in four growth-impaired children[21]. Subsequently, others have confirmed these results in hospitalized[22] and ambulatory patients[29]. More recently, the form of nutrition support has emphasized the enteral route. Similar benefits in improving growth velocity occur after formula supplements, either oral[23,27] or by nocturnal nasogastric infusion, on a regular[25,26,37] or intermittent[28] schedule.

The method of nutrition support for an individual patient must take into account the severity of disease activity and symptoms. Morin *et al.* have shown that, for improved growth to continue after a four-week period of elemental formula infusion, disease activity must be controlled so that adequate calorie intake is maintained[26].

Controversy exists concerning recommendations to supply the calories necessary to reverse growth failure. We found that increasing calorie intake from 54% to 91% of the RDA was sufficient to initiate normal growth[23]; others[25,37] have suggested exceeding the RDA by 30–50%. Recommendations[21-23,25-29,37,38] for calorie intake based on body weight range from 50 to 93 kcal kg^{-1} day^{-1}.

In our patients, providing 91% of the RDA for age and sex was equivalent to 75 kcal kg^{-1} day^{-1}. The higher energy intake per kilogram body weight is, at least in part, a reflection of the weight loss most of these children have experienced.

Surgical resection should be considered for children whose impaired growth does not respond to medical therapy with nutrition support as described above. This is particularly indicated for patients with localized Crohn's disease and those with chronic non-specific ulcerative colitis. Results are best when surgery is performed in the prepubertal period and, in patients with Crohn's disease, when disease recurrence is delayed.[39,40]

SUMMARY

The clinical diversity in paediatric patients with Crohn's disease and chronic non-specific ulcerative colitis is great as described in the foregoing discussion. Attention to growth rate is an important corollary to the management of both diseases.

The challenge for paediatric gastroenterologists entrusted with the care of these children is to maintain long-term control of disease activity to ensure adequate nutrient intake during the period of linear growth. We have shown that it may take several years after diagnosis for a growth-impaired child to achieve his/her pre-illness height percentile[23]. Therapeutic intervention should consider individualized drug therapy (including alternate-day prednisone administration; immunosuppressive drugs, such as azathioprine/6-mercaptopurine and, possibly, cyclosporine); providing adequate nutrition support (oral formulae, nasogastric feeding, home parenteral nutrition); timing of surgery and psychological support.

References

1. Barton, J.R., Gillon, S. and Ferguson, A. (1989). Incidence of inflammatory bowel disease in Scottish children between 1968 and 1983: marginal fall in ulcerative colitis, three-fold rise in Crohn's disease. *Gut*, **30**, 618–622
2. Farmer, R.G. and Michener, W.M. (1979). Prognosis of Crohn's disease with onset in childhood or adolescence. *Dig. Dis. Sci.*, **24**, 752–757
3. Michener, W.M., Whelan, G., Greenstreet, R.L. and Farmer, R.G. (1982). Comparison of the clinical features of Crohn's disease and ulcerative colitis with onset in childhood or adolescence. *Cleveland Clin. Q.*, **49**, 13–16
4. Calkins, B.H. and Mendeloff, A.I. (1986). Epidemiology of inflammatory bowel disease. *Epidemiol. Rev.*, **8**, 60–91
5. Gilat, T. and Langman, M.J.S. (1987). Childhood factors in ulcerative colitis and Crohn's disease: an international cooperative study. *Scand. J. Gastroenterol.*, **22**, 1009–1024
6. Mayer, L. and Shlien, R. (1987). Evidence for function of Ia molecules on gut eipthelial cells in man. *J. Exp. Med.*, **166**, 1471–1483
7. Mayer, L. and Eisenhardt, D. (1987). Lack of induction of suppressor T cells by gut epithelial cells from patients with inflammatory bowel disease. The primary defect? (Abstract) *Gastroenterology*, **92**, 1524
8. MacDermott, R.P. (1987). Expression of human immunoglobulin G subclasses in inflammatory bowel diseases. *Gastroenterology*, **93**, 1127–1134
9. Hirata, I., Berrivi, G., Austin, L.L., Keren, D.F. and Dobbins, W.O. III. (1986). Induction of HLA-DR antigens on colonic epithelial cells in inflammatory bowel disease. *Dig. Dis. Sci.*, **31**, 593–603
10. Markowitz, J., Daum, F., Aiges, H., Kahn, E., Silverberg, M. and Fisher, S.E. (1984). Perianal disease in children and adolescents with Crohn's disease. *Gastroenterology*, **86**, 829–833
11. Michener, W.M., Farmer, R.G. and Mortimer, E.A. (1979). Long-term prognosis of ulcerative colitis with onset in childhood and adolescence. *J. Clin. Gastroenterol.*, **1**, 301–305
12. Mir-Madhjessi, S.H., Michener, W.M. and Farmer, R.G. (1986). Course and prognosis of idiopathic ulcerative proctosigmoiditis in young patients. *J. Pediatr. Gastroenterol. Nutr.*, **5**, 570–575
13. Burbige, E.J., Huang, S.S. and Bayless, T.M. (1975). Clinical manifestations of Crohn's disease in children and adolescents. *Pediatrics*, **55**, 866–871
14. Passo, M.H., Fitzgerald, J.F. and Brandt, K.D. (1986). Arthritis associated with inflammatory bowel disease: relationship of joint disease to activity and severity of bowel lesion. *Dig. Dis. Sci.*, **31**, 492–497
15. Greenstein, A.J., Sachar, D.B., Pucillo, A., Vassiliades, G., Smith, H., Kreel, I., Geller, S.A., Janowitz, H.D. and Aufses, A.H. (1979). The extra-intestinal complications of Crohn's disease and ulcerative colitis: a study of 700 patients. *Medicine*, **55**, 401–412
16. Kirschner, B.S. and Samowitz, W.S. (1986). Secondary amyloidosis in Crohn's disease of childhood. *J. Pediatr. Gastroenterol. Nutr.*, **5**, 816–821
17. Paradis, K., Bernstein, M.L. and Adelson, J.W. (1985). Thrombosis as a complication of inflammatory bowel disease in children; a report of four cases. *J. Pediatr. Gastroenterol. Nutr.*, **4**, 659–662
18. Markowitz, R.L., Ment, L.R. and Gryboski, J.D. (1989). Cerebral thromboembolic disease in pediatric and adult inflammatory bowel disease: case report and review of the literature. *J. Pediatr. Gastroenterol. Nutr.*, **8**, 413–420
19. Kirschner, B.S., Voinchet, O. and Rosenberg, I.H. (1978). Growth retardation in inflammatory bowel disease. *Gastroenterology*, **75**, 504–511
20. Kanof, M.E., Lake, A.M. and Bayless, T.M. (1988). Decreased height velocity in children and adolescents before the diagnosis of Crohn's disease. *Gastroenterology*, **95**, 1523–1527
21. Layden, T., Rosenberg, J., Nemchausky, B., Elson, C. and Rosenberg, I. (1976). Reversal of growth arrest in adolescents with Crohn's disease after parenteral alimentation.

Gastroenterology, **70**, 1017–1026
22. Kelts, D.G., Grand, R.J., Shen, G., Watkins, J.B., Werlin, S.L. and Boehme, C. (1979). Nutritional basis of growth failure in children and adolescents with Crohn's disease. *Gastroenterology*, **76**, 720–727
23. Kirschner, B.S., Klich, J.R., Kalman, S.S., deFavaro, M.V. and Rosenberg, I.H. (1981). Reversal of growth retardation in Crohn's disease with therapy emphasizing oral nutritional restitution. *Gastroenterology*, **80**, 10–15
24. Motil, K.J., Altschuler, S.I. and Grand, R.J. (1985). Mineral balance during nutritional supplementation in adolescents with Crohn's disease and growth failure. *J. Pediatr.*, **107**, 473–479
25. Motil, K.J., Grand, R.J., Maletskos, C.J. and Young, V.R. (1982). The effect of disease, drug and diet on whole body protein metabolism in adolescents with Crohn's disease and growth failure. *J. Pediatr.*, **101**, 345–351
26. Morin, C.L., Roulet, M. and Weber, A. (1980). Continuous elemental enteral alimentation in children with Crohn's disease and growth failure. *Gastroenterology*, **79**, 1205–1210
27. O'Morain, C., Segal, A., Levi, A.J. and Valman, H.B. (1983). Elemental diet in acute Crohn's disease. *Arch. Dis. Child.*, **53**, 44–47
28. Belli, D.C., Seidman, E., Bouthillier, L., Weber, A.H., Roy, C.C., Pletincx, M., Beaulieu, M. and Morin, C.L. (1988). Chronic intermittent elemental diet improves growth failure in children with Crohn's disease. *Gastroenterology*, **94**, 603–610
29. Strobel, C.T., Byrne, W.J. and Ament, M.E. (1979). Home parenteral nutrition in children with Crohn's disease: an effective management alternative. *Gastroenterology*, **77**, 272–279
30. Kirschner, B.S., Schoeller, D.A. and Sutton, M.M. (1984). Measurement of energy expenditure (EE) in adolescents with Crohn's disease (C.D.) using doubly-labelled water. (Abstract) *Gastroenterology*, **86**, 1136
31. Gotlin, E.W. and Dubois, R.S. (1973). Nyctohemeral growth hormone levels in children with growth retardation and inflammatory bowel disease. *Gut*, **14**, 191–195
32. Tenore, R.L., Berman, W.F., Parks, J.S. and Bongiovanni, A.M. (1977). Basal and stimulated growth hormone concentrations in inflammatory bowel disease. *J. Clin. Endocrinol. Metab.*, **44**, 622–628
33. Farthing, M.J.G., Campbell, C.A., Walker-Smith, J., Edwards, C.R.W., Rees, L.H. and Dawson, A.M. (1981). Nocturnal growth hormone and gonadotropin secretion in growth retarded children with Crohn's disease. *Gut*, **22**, 933–938
34. Kirschner, B.S. and Sutton, M.M. (1986). Somatomedin-C level in growth-impaired children and adolescents with chronic inflammatory bowel disease. *Gastroenterology*, **91**, 830–836
35. Phillips, L.S. and Young, H.S. (1976). Nutrition and somatomedin, I. Effect of fasting and refeeding on serum somatomedin activity and cartilage growth activity in rats. *Endocrinology*, **99**, 304–314
36. Chong, S.K.F., Grossman, A., Walker-Smith, J.A. and Rees, L.H. (1984). Endocrine dysfunction in children with Crohn's disease. *J. Pediatr. Gastroenterol. Nutr.*, **3**, 529–534
37. Navarro, J., Vargas, J., Cezard, J.P., Charritat, J.L. and Polonovski, C. (1982), Prolonged constant rate elemental enteral nutrition in Crohn's disease. *J. Pediatr. Gastroenterol. Nutr.*, **1**, 541–546
38. Kirschner, B.S. (1988). Enteral nutrition in inflammatory bowel disease. In *Report of the 94th Ross Conference on Pediatric Research, Enteral Feeding: Scientific Basis and Clinical Applications*. pp. 103–109. (Ohio: Ross Laboratories)
39. Homer, D.R., Grand, R.J. and Colodny, A.H. (1977). Growth course and prognosis after surgery for Crohn's disease. *Pediatrics*, **59**, 717–725
40. Wesson, D.E. and Schandling, B. (1981). Results of bowel resection for Crohn's disease in the young. *J. Pediatr. Surg.*, **16**, 449–452

4
Evaluation of endoscopic findings in Crohn's disease of childhood and adolescence

M. BURDELSKI, H.-G. POSSELT, M. BECKER, R.-M. BERTELE-HARMS, B. RODECK, P.-F. HOYER and P. SCHMITZ-MOORMANN

INTRODUCTION

Diagnostic criteria in Crohn's disease are well established in adults as far as radiological, histological and endoscopic criteria are concerned[1-4]. Most of these criteria have been developed for therapeutic studies. That is why they are very strict and do not stick to early signs of the disease. Up to now, only the radiological and histological criteria of the adult studies have been applied for diagnostic purposes in children and adolescents[5-7]. These studies have shown that many paediatric patients do not fulfil radiological or histological criteria at the initial examination[5-10].

In the meantime, endoscopy has proved to be an important diagnostic tool in acute and chronic inflammatory bowel disease of infancy and childhood[11,12]. Using the endoscopic expertise of four paediatric centres, a prospective multicentre study was designed in order to evaluate the endoscopic findings in the upper and lower gastrointestinal tract in children and adolescents suffering from either radiologically or histologically proven non-treated Crohn's disease (CD). The aims of this study were: (1) to document the endoscopic visible features of CD at this stage of the disease; (2) to evaluate endoscopic criteria by comparing them with radiological and histological ones; and (3) to investigate to which extent endoscopic features of CD may be regarded as early signs of this disease.

PATIENTS AND METHODS

From 1982 to 1986, all patients with initial presentation of chronic inflammatory bowel disease at the Children's Hospitals of Bonn, Frankfurt, Hannover and Munich were investigated according to an identical examination protocol. This protocol included complete colonoscopy and histology of biopsies and radiology of the small bowel. The endoscopic findings were documented by the four local endoscopists. The documentation forms were transferred later to one centre for statistical analysis. The documentation scheme counted the occurrence of defined lesions (Figure 1) per intestinal segment, the segments being defined as rectum/sigmoid/descending/transverse/ascending colon and caecum/oesophagus/stomach/duodenum. Thus, the analysis of the endoscopic findings yields a qualitative evaluation of the endoscopic features of CD.

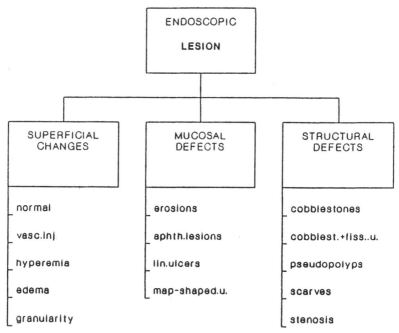

Figure 1 Classification of endoscopic lesions in small and large bowel endoscopy. Abbreviations: vasc. inj. = vascular injection; aphth. lesions = aphthoid lesions; lin, ulcers = linear ulcers; u. = ulcers; fiss. = fissural

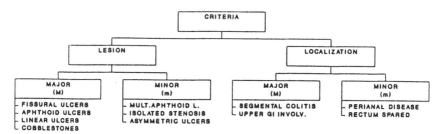

Figure 2 Endoscopic criteria used in this study, divided in major (M) and minor (m) lesions and localizations. Abbreviation: involv. = involvement. The diagnosis was accepted with at least MMm or Mmmm

Serial biopsies taken during endoscopy were examined by the reference pathologist of the study. The work-up of these biopsies was extensive, using up to 100 serial lamination steps per biopsy. The X-ray films were seen and evaluated by four reference radiologists of the study referring to established criteria[8,9]. The endoscopic criteria were adapted to adult criteria[2,13,14]. The only modification was the acceptance of pronounced upper gastrointestinal involvement as a major criterion (Figure 2). CD was diagnosed endoscopically if 2 major plus 1 minor or 1 major plus 3 minor criteria were observed. Patients with chronic inflammatory bowel disease different from CD according to both radiological and histological findings were taken as controls.

RESULTS

A total of 92 patients were accepted as suffering from CD by radiological and/or histological criteria by means of small bowel radiology and complete colonoscopy. In a subpopulation of 62 patients, a complete upper gastrointestinal endoscopy was available. An additional 8 patients had insufficient documentation of endoscopic lesions for statistical analysis but sufficient for evaluation of endoscopic criteria. 13 patients served as controls after CD had been excluded.

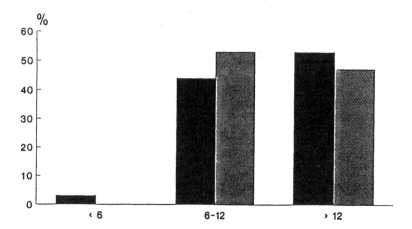

Figure 3 Age distribution in percent of patients with proven Crohn's disease (■) and controls (Cd excluded, ▨) in years

Patients with CD were aged between 4 and 18 years, the majority being older than 12 years. In the group of non-CD patients, there were patients between 6 and 16 years of age (Figure 3).

The localization of the different endoscopic lesions of the upper gastrointestinal tract and of the colon is shown in Figure 4. In the upper gastrointestinal tract, there was a predominance of gastric lesions which

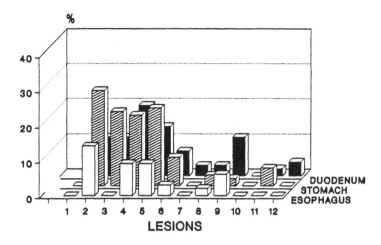

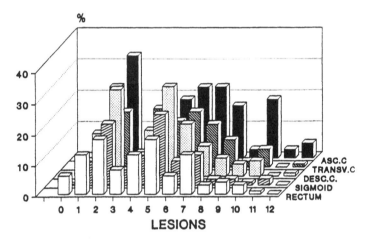

Figure 4 Results of qualitative analysis of endoscopic lesions in the upper gastrointestinal tract (upper part, n = 62) and the colon (lower part, n = 92). 0 = injection; 2= hyperaemia; 3 = oedema; 4 = granularity; 5 = erosion; 6 = aphthoid lesion; 7 = linear ulcer; 8 = map-shaped ulcer; 9 = cobblestone + fissural ulcer; 10 = cobblestone; 11 = pseudopolyp; 12 = scarve; 13 = stenosis

were observed in more than 20% of patients. Superficial lesions, like hyperaemia, oedema, granularity, erosions and aphthoid lesions, were the most frequent features, whereas structural defects, such as cobblestones and stenosis, were only rare findings in the duodenum. Most of the lesions showed a patchy distribution or were observed as isolated lesions.

As far as the lesions in the large bowel are concerned, superficial lesions, such as hyperaemia, oedema, granularity and aphthous lesions, were observed in the distal colon only as frequently as in the stomach. Ulcerations, cobblestones, pseudopolyps, scarves and stenosis, however, showed a remarkable shift to the right colon. There was a strong segmental character of the inflammatory lesions throughout the colon, which is shown in Figure 5. The activity of the inflammatory process was related to increasing numbers of different lesions per segment. In patients with CD, the most active site of the disease was observed in the right colon (Figure 5).

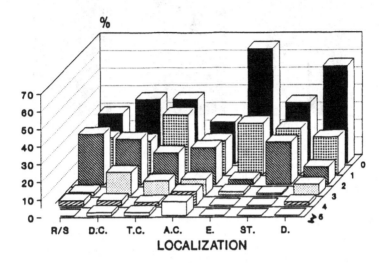

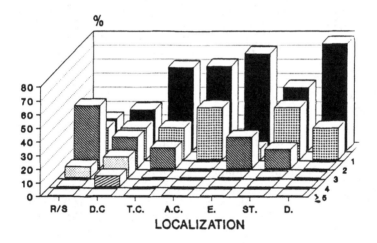

Figure 5 Frequencies of different endoscopic lesions in paediatric patients with Crohn's disease (upper) and patients with excluded Crohn's disease (lower). R/S = rectosigmoid; D.C. = descending colon; T.C. = transverse colon; A.C. = ascending colon; E = oesophagus; ST. = stomach; D. = duodenum. 0 = lesion free; 1–5 = numbers of different kinds of endoscopic lesions per segment

The diagnostic sensitivity and specificity of histology, radiology and endoscopy based on the diagnostic criteria of each method was calculated for 70 patients suffering from CD and 13 patients with non-CD. The

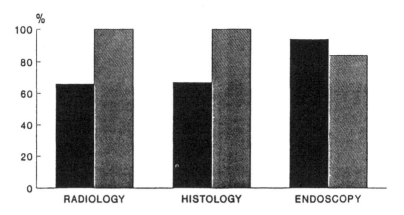

Figure 6 Diagnostic sensitivity (■) and specificity (▨) of radiological, histological and endoscopic criteria in patients with Crohn's disease (n = 100) and patients with chronic inflammatory bowel disease other than Crohn's disease (n = 13)

diagnostic sensitivity was highest in endoscopy, the diagnostic specificity, on the other hand, was below that of radiology and histology (Figure 6). Corresponding positive criteria in radiology, histology and endoscopy were only observed in 19% of patients. Positive histological findings were documented in 67% and positive radiological findings in 60% of the cases. 25% of patients had positive histological criteria in the upper gastrointestinal tract. In the control group, there were all negative radiological and histological findings; 2 of these patients, however, fulfilled the endoscopic criteria of CD.

DISCUSSION

This study yields information about qualitative features of endoscopically visible lesions in the upper and lower gastrointestinal tract of children and adolescents with chronic inflammatory bowel disease. The upper gastrointestinal tract was found to be involved in Crohn's disease in more than 20% of the patients studied, the most significant localization being the stomach. This finding is surprising since there are no such results reported so far[15-17]. An involvement to such an extent has been described in adult patients only if upper gastrointestinal endoscopy was performed as obligatory examination[18]. In studies with facultative upper gastrointestinal endoscopy, the frequency of gastric lesions in CD is much lower[1,14]. There are comparable endoscopic large bowel findings in paediatric and adult patients too. The right and the descending colon are the most important localizations in both age groups[2]. The difference between children and adults is mainly the different degree of severity: in children there is a predominance of superficial lesions, like erosions and aphthoid lesions, which seem to change into deep mucosal defects in adults[2,19]. These severe mucosal lesions are observed in children and adolescents in the right colon only[4-6]. This finding might have been suspected from the radiological findings in paediatric CD[8]. The distribution of endoscopically detectable lesions is a pronounced segmental one.

These findings suggest that, in children and adolescents with suspected chronic inflammatory bowel disease, upper gastrointestinal endoscopy and complete colonoscopy should be performed routinely in order to optimize the diagnostic efficacy. The endoscopic criteria used in this study allowed a safe endoscopic diagnosis of CD. The diagnostic sensitivity and specificity achieved by these criteria seem to be acceptable especially in order to diagnose CD at an early stage. Taking the pronounced gastrointestinal involvement as a major endoscopic criterion seems to be reasonable if the findings of the stomach and duodenum are considered. In comparison, our own criteria may be regarded as more distinctive[10,15-17].

The major advantage of endoscopy in the diagnostic approach to chronic inflammatory bowel disease is the opportunity to obtain histological examinations of biopsies taken from all examined gastrointestinal segments. 40% of diagnosed CD would have been missed without endoscopy and histology since small bowel radiology was not conclusive. This can only be done, however, if the histological work-up of the biopsies is as extensive as that performed in our study[9]. Routine histology will not allow diagnosis of CD to the same extent as the laminary section technique. Provided that these endoscopic criteria and this histological work-up are used, endoscopy and histology will enable the desirable aim of early diagnosis of Crohn's disease in children and adults.

Acknowledgement

This study was part of the study 'Morbus Crohn beim Kind' and supported by the Stiftung Volkswagenwerk, AZ: I-36 646.

References

1. Lind, E., Fausa, O., Elgjo, K. and Gjone, E. (1985). Crohn's disease – diagnostic procedures and problems. *Scand. J. Gastroenterol.*, **20**, 660–664
2. Lorenz-Meyer, H., Malchow, H., Miller, B., Stock, H. and Brandes, J.W. (1985). European Cooperative Crohn's Disease Study (ECCDS): colonoscopy. *Digestion*, **31**, 109–119
3. Malchow, H. and Daiss, W. (1984). Diagnostik des M. Crohn. *Dtsch. M. Wschr.*, **109**, 1770–1775
4. Myrem, J., Bouchier, I.A.D., Watkinson, G. and Softley, A. (1984). The OMGE Multinational Inflammatory Bowel Disease Survey. 1972–1982. *Scand. J. Gastroenterol.*, **95** (Suppl.), 1–27
5. Bender, S.W. (1977). Crohn's disease in children: initial symptomatology. *Acta Paediatr. Belg.*, **30**, 193
6. Bender, S.W., Kirchmann, H. and Posselt, H-G. (1986). Morbus Crohn im Kindesalter. *Wien. Klin. Wochenschr.*, **16**, 520–527
7. Hauke, H, Lassrich, M.A. and Ball, F. (1978). Ergebnisse einer radiologischen Studie bei M. Crohn im Kindesalter. *Radiologe*, **18**, 199–207
8. Ball, F., Hauke, H., Lassrich, M.A., Schuster, W., Reither, M. and Stöver, V. (1990). Radiologic evaluation of 501 pediatric patients with Crohn's disease – Localization, extent and severity of radiological changes. *Fortschr. Röntgenstr.* (planned to submit)

9. Schmitz-Moormann, P. and Schaeg, M. (1990). Histology of the lower intestinal tract in Crohn's disease in children and adolescents. *Pathol. Res. Pract.* (submitted)

10. Dubois, R.S., Rothschild, J., Silverman, A. and Sabra, A. (1978). The varied manifestation of Crohn's disease in children and adolescents. *Am. J. Gastroenterol.*, 1978, **69**, 203–211

11. Burdelski, M. and Huchzermeyer, H. (Eds.). (1981). *Gastrointestinale Endoskopie im Kindesalter.* (Berlin, Heidelberg, New York: Springer)

12. Cadranel, S., Rodesch, P., Peckos, J.P. and Cremer, M. (1977). Fiberendoscopy of the gastrointestinal tract in children. *Am. J. Dis. Child.*, **131**, 41–45

13. Malchow, H., Ewe, K., Brandes, J.W., Goebell, H., Ehms, H., Sommer, H. and Jerdinsky, H. (1984). European Cooperative Crohn's Disease Study (ECCDS). Results of drug treatment. *Gastroenterology*, **86**, 249–266

14. Lind, E., Fausa, O., Elgjo, K. and Gjone, E. (1985). Crohn's disease. Clinical manifestations. *Scand. J. Gastroenterol.*, **20**, 665–670

15. Chong, S.K.F. and Walker-Smith, J.A. (1982). Chronic inflammatory bowel disease in the young. *Compr. Ther.*, **8**, 27–34

16. Chong, S.K.F., Blackshaw, A.J., Boyle, S., Williams, C.B. and Walker-Smith, J.A. (1985). Histological diagnosis of chronic inflammatory bowel disease in childhood. *Gut.*, **8**, 55–59

17. O'Donoghue, D.P. and Dawson, A.M. (1977). Crohn's disease in childhood. *Arch. Dis. Child.*, **52**, 627–632

18. Kurtz, B., Steinhardt, H.J. and Malchow, H. (1982). M. Crohn des oberen Gastrointestinaltraktes im radiologischen und endoskopischen Bild. *Fortschr. Röntgenstr.*, **136**, 124–128

19. Steinhardt, H.J., Loeschke, K., Kasper, H., Holtmüller, H.H. and Schäfter, H. (1985). European Cooperative Crohn's Disease Study (ECCDS). Clinical features and natural history. *Digestion*, **31**, 97–108

5
Diagnostic imaging in inflammatory bowel disease in paediatric patients

C.P. FLIEGEL and F. HADZISELIMOVIC

Barium radiography and endoscopy are the primary methods for evaluation of inflammatory bowel disease (IBD) in children[1]. These two methods are sufficient for detection of mucosal lesions of the entire gastrointestinal tract with the exception of those parts of the small bowel which are not accessible for the endoscope. The two methods, however, cannot reliably detect extraluminal lesions and frequently cannot determine the thickness of the bowel wall. This applies to primary manifestations as well as complications of IBD, such as abscess, fistulae, perirectal disease, mesenteric disease, bone involvement, hepatobiliary complications, and complications of the urinary tract. For all these questions, the cross-sectional imaging modalities, especially ultrasound and computerized tomography, provide additional answers. These two methods are also helpful in differentiating the two main entities of inflammatory bowel disease, namely Crohn's disease and ulcerative colitis. This is true for approximately 85% of all cases leaving out those patients with so-called indeterminate colitis.

In the following presentation, we would like to give an outline of the relevant findings in selected cases from our own patients and present our current approach to the diagnosis of inflammatory bowel disease on first presentation and on follow-up studies and complications.

ULCERATIVE COLITIS

In this disease, computerized tomography (CT) is helpful only in cases of long duration. Computerized tomography will show bowel wall thickness[2] greater than 3 mm but usually less than 10 mm. The colon wall often has inhomogeneous attenuation with regions of fat density.

A typical case of long-standing ulcerative colitis is shown in Figure 1a–d. Rectal and perirectal changes in ulcerative colitis result in the typical target appearance of the rectum produced by alternating zones of soft-tissue

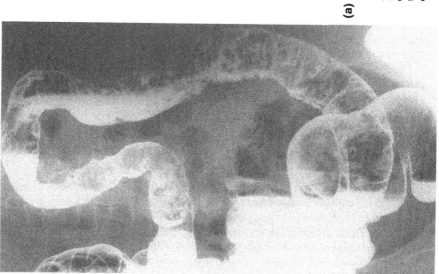

(a)

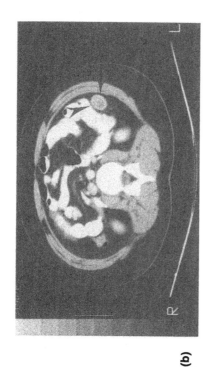
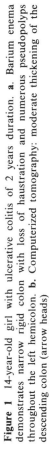

(b)

Figure 1 14-year-old girl with ulcerative colitis of 2 years duration. **a.** Barium enema demonstrates narrow rigid colon with loss of haustration and numerous pseudopolyps throughout the left hemicolon. **b.** Computerized tomography: moderate thickening of the descending colon (arrow heads)

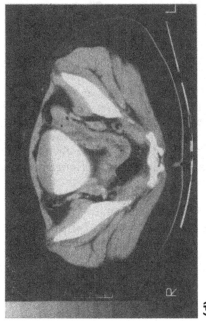

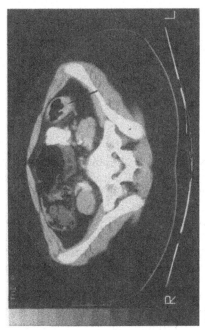

Figure 1 continued **c.** Same examination at the level of S_1 demonstrates an irregular thickening of the colon wall with pseudopolyp formation (arrow). Irregular attenuation of bowel wall density. **d.** CT cut at the level of the bladder demonstrates a segment of the sigmoid colon with narrow lumen and irregular thickening of the wall indicating severe involvement by ulcerative colitis

77

density, fat density and again soft-tissue density. The lumen is usually narrow whereas the presacral space is increased.

CROHN'S DISEASE

In Crohn's disease, bowel wall thickening can be massive, up to 20 mm and more in the late stages. In the early stages, bowel wall thickening[2] may be completely absent or between 4 and 10 mm. In a proven case of Crohn's disease, intestinal wall thickness is a good indicator for the activity of the disease, and, therefore, CT imaging as well as ultrasound are very useful in follow-up studies under medical treatment to determine the degree of activity.

Mesenteric disease, as seen by CT, consists of fatty infiltration, thickening of the mesentery and lymph node proliferation.

A typical case of Crohn's disease with ileocaecal involvement is shown in Figure 2a and b. A recently observed complication in Crohn's disease is transient intussusception in patients with long-standing disease and acute episodes of abdominal pain. It was first described by Knowle[2] and was also observed in one of our patients (Figure 3). The significance of the findings is two-fold:

1. It explains the acute abdominal pain, and
2. It does not need surgical intervention; once identified by CT, it will subside spontaneously.

Ultrasound examination can partially replace CT especially in determining the thickness of the terminal ileum as demonstrated in Figure 4a and b in a 9-year-old patient where Crohn's disease was clinically suspected and demonstrated by ultrasound and subsequent small bowel barium study.

DISCUSSION

A comparative study by Greenstein[3] between CT and barium examinations in patients with Crohn's disease indicated that CT was superior to barium in the diagnosis of mesenteric disease, enterovesical fistula, abscess in unusual location, especially psoasabscess, and bone involvement.

In the same study, barium was superior to CT in cases with enterofistulae, strictures and recurrent disease after surgery. The study was done in 43 adult patients and therefore is only of limited significance for paediatric patients, but it probably can be considered a useful guideline for younger patients as well.

Differentiation of Crohn's disease and ulcerative colitis is usually possible on the grounds of clinical, laboratory, endoscopic and conventional roentgen findings. When CT and ultrasound findings are used as additional criteria, the separation of the two entities becomes more reliable. The main CT findings of the two entities are listed in Table 1.

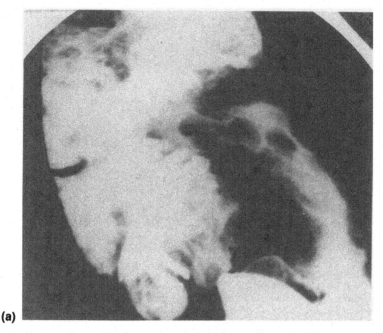

(a)

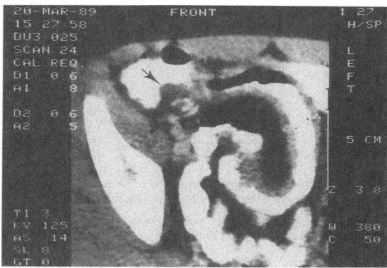

(b)

Figure 2 13-year-old boy with suspicion of Crohn's disease. **a.** Barium study shows loss of normal mucosal pattern of the terminal ileum, thickening of the ileocaecal valve and a relatively mild degree of cobblestone pattern. **b.** CT examination of the ileocaecal area showing a prominent ileocaecal valve (arrow). Moderate thickening of the wall of the terminal ileum (6 mm). Both studies are typical for Crohn's disease of relatively short duration

Taking into consideration the present state of the literature[4,5] and our own experience with 12 recent cases of IBD, we recommend the following approach for diagnostic work-up:

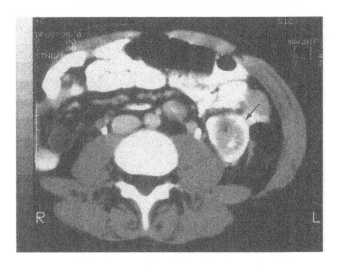

Figure 3 14-year-old boy with long-standing Crohn's disease under conservative treatment and acute onset of lower abdominal pain. CT scan demonstrates a target lesion in the left lower quadrant consisting of an outer rim of contrast material (arrow), an intermediate zone of bowel wall density and a central spot of contrast and air. The findings are typical for intussusception which turned out to be of transient nature

Table 1 Crohn's disease vs. ulcerative colitis as seen by CT

Feature	Crohn's disease	Ulcerative colitis
Bowel wall	>10 mm	<10 mm
Wall density	Homogeneous	Inhomogeneous
Rectum	Fistulae	Target sign
Abscess	Common	Rare or absent
Mesentery	LN + thickening	Normal
Fistulae	Common	Rare
Intussusception	Yes	No

LN = lymph node proliferation

1. In the early stages of the disease: endoscopy combined with barium studies of the gastrointestinal tract, including the ileocaecal area.

2. In long-standing inflammatory bowel disease including complications: ultrasound and computerized tomography.

CONCLUSION

CT and ultrasound have been of additional value in IBD for the following reasons:

1. Better delineation of mural and extramural disease,
2. More confident separation of Crohn's disease and ulcerative colitis,
3. Reliable evaluation of response to medical treatment by monitoring wall thickness of the involved segments of bowel,

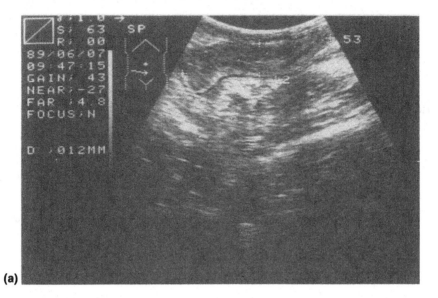

(a)

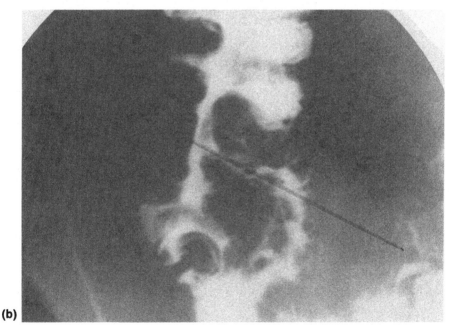

(b)

Figure 4 9-year-old boy with great weight loss, anaemia and lower abdominal pain. **a.** Initial ultrasound study demonstrates a distal loop of small bowel with marked thickening of the wall (6 mm). **b.** Barium study, spot film of ileocaecal area demonstrating typical changes of Crohn's disease with transverse and longitudinal fissures, cobblestone pattern and massive thickening of ileocaecal valve and similar changes of the caecum. The transverse line indicates the sectional plane during the ultrasound examination. Follow-up ultrasound in this patient after 4 months of medical treatment showed an identical degree of bowel wall thickening consistent with unsatisfactory response to medical treatment

4. Preoperative assistance in making a decision for or against colectomy in ulcerative colitis by evaluation of the terminal ileum to rule out Crohn's disease.

References

1. Gore, R. (1989). CT of inflammatory bowel disease. *Radiol. Clin. N. Am.*, **27**, 4, 717–729
2. Knowles, M. (1989). Transient intussusception in Crohn disease: CT evaluation. *Radiology*, **170**, 814
3. Greenstein, S. (1987). Computed tomography vs barium studies in the acutely symptomatic patient with Crohn disease. *J. Comput. Assist. Tomograph.*, **11**, 6, 1009–1016
4. Riddlesberger, M.M. (1985). CT of complicated inflammatory bowel disease in children. *Ped. Radiol.*, **15**, 384–387
5. Siegel, M.J. (1988). Small bowel disease in children: Diagnosis with CT. *Ped. Radiol.*, **169**, 127–130
6. Stringer, D. (1987). Imaging inflammatory bowel disease in the pediatric patient. *Radiol. Clin. N. Am.*, **25**, 1, 93–113

6
Lymphocyte subsets in Crohn's disease

B. RODECK, M.R. HADAM and M. BURDELSKI

INTRODUCTION

The aetiology of Crohn's disease remains unresolved, though it is generally accepted that the immune system may be involved in its pathogenesis. Peripheral blood lymphocytes have been the starting point for many investigations of immune function, mainly due to easy accessibility. However, these studies have yielded conflicting results concerning the number and function of immunocytes in peripheral blood[1]. The development of monoclonal antibody-based techniques has provided a much closer insight into the lymphocyte subsets involved in immune regulation and effector responses. Thus, monoclonal antibodies can be used to define several functionally distinct classes of T lymphocytes, such as helper/inducer (CD4-positive) or suppressor/cytotoxic (CD8-positive) T lymphocytes. Using monoclonal antibodies to these markers, Selby and Jewel[2] and Yuan[3] found no significant differences in the proportion of circulating T lymphocytes or their subsets between Crohn's disease patients and controls. Recently, the antigen receptor on T lymphoctyes has been identified as a two-chain structure whose expression is linked to the CD3-antigen complex. Antigen recognition by most T cells is accomplished by a heterodimeric receptor protein termed TCR2 composed of disulfide-linked α and β chains[4]. On some rare T lymphocytes which express CD3 without TCR2, a second T cell receptor, distinct from TCR2, was discovered. This receptor (TCR1) consists of two proteins (γ,δ) which may or may not be disulfide linked[5]. Less than 9% of CD3-positive lymphocytes in human peripheral blood express this receptor. Recently, monoclonal antibodies against both TCR1[6] and TCR2[7] have become available which allow direct quantification of TCR subtypes in patients' blood samples.

Several years ago, we found in a few patients with Crohn's disease increased numbers of CD3+CD4−CD8− cells, a phenotype which is now considered characteristic for TCR1-bearing cells. Based on these observations, we initiated a prospective study on the distribution of T cell receptors in paediatric patients with Crohn's disease.

Materials and methods – patients

Sixty-two paediatric patients with Crohn's disease were examined. The diagnosis of Crohn's disease was established according to the diagnostic criteria of the Pediatric Crohn's Disease Study Group[8]. Mean age was 15.9 years (range 7.3–23.1); 35 patients were male, 27 female. Disease activity was assessed using a paediatric Crohn's disease activity index as proposed by Harms *et al.*[9]. Mononuclear cell suspensions were prepared from fresh peripheral blood samples by standard density gradient centrifugation. Indirect immunofluorescence labelling was performed using appropriate monoclonal antibodies and fluorescein-labelled $F(ab')_2$-fragments of goat-anti-mouse-immunoglobulin antibodies (Jackson Immunosearch) as second step reagents. Lymphocyte subsets were evaluated on a fluorescence-activated cell sorter (FACS 440) after gating on lymphocytes only. Routinely CD3, TCR2, CD8, CD4, CD5, CD22 and CD71 antibodies were employed. In informative cases, an antibody against TCR1 (TCRδ1, T Cell Sciences) was used in addition.

RESULTS

In our prospective study on paediatric patients with Morbus Crohn, we determined the relative number of TCR1-bearing lymphocytes consecutively up to 847 days; mean observation period was 446 days. Determinations were usually performed every 4 months; altogether, 455 blood samples were evaluated.

The 90th percentile of TCR1-bearing lymphocytes in the peripheral blood of normal blood donors and a control group consisting of unselected other patients (except Morbus Crohn) is below 9% of all lymphocytes (n = 435; Figure 1). In 15 out of 62 patients with paediatric Morbus Crohn, more than 12% of all T lymphocytes were found to express TCR1 on at least two occasions. As is readily apparent from Figure 1, the 90th percentile is only reached at 16% TCR1-bearing cells in patients with Morbus Crohn. The corresponding values for the 95th percentile are <12% TCR1 for the control group versus 24% TCR1-bearing lymphocytes in the patients. Interestingly, the initial slope of both percentile distributions is virtually identical, pointing to a similar proportion of lymphocytes which are low or negative for TCR1 both in patients and controls. Plotting the differential of both curves yields a broad maximum at 12% TCR1 (not shown).

In addition, we tried to correlate both absolute number and percentage of TCR1-positive lymphocytes with the paediatric Crohn's disease activity index. In only a few patients, we found moderate correlation during the course of the disease.

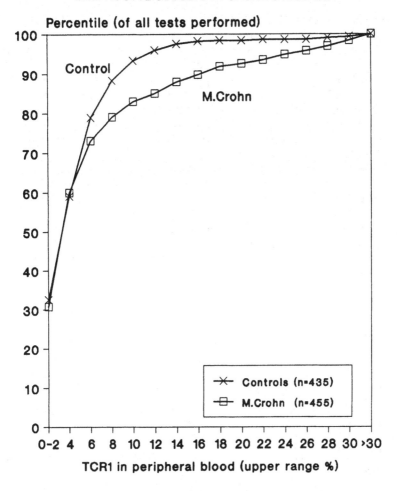

Figure 1 TCR1 in controls and paediatric Morbus Crohn

DISCUSSION

In this study, we have investigated prospectively the distribution of T lymphocytes expressing one form of the T cell receptor (TCR1) in children and adolescents suffering from Crohn's disease. This type of receptor is normally found in a minority of peripheral blood T lymphocytes only. We describe here a subset of patients which have significantly more circulating T lymphocytes with TCR1 compared with a control group. Similar observations have not been reported so far. Our results are supported by Elson *et al*.[10], who investigated two patients with Morbus Crohn and abnormal suppressor cell activity. Careful review of their patients' peripheral-blood T-lymphocyte phenotype reveals a marked expansion of CD3+CD4-CD8- T lymphoctyes which is now considered characteristic for TCR1-positive cells. Their findings may also point to a functional role of this novel T-cell subset. Interestingly, we found elevated levels of TCR1 cells in only 24% of our case. Careful examination of case histories did not reveal clear correlations of our laboratory findings with clinical parameters. Variables investigated included age, sex, duration of disease, mode and duration of therapy. However, in all patients with elevated TCR1, the areas of intestinal inflammation were found to be primarily localized in the colon. As cells bearing TCR1 are selectively found as intraepithelial lymphocytes in the intestinal wall of mice[11], our findings – albeit relating to peripheral blood – may reveal a functional role of TCR1-bearing T cells in human gastrointestinal physiology.

SUMMARY

We describe a subgroup of paediatric patients suffering from Crohn's disease that show abnormally high numbers of TCR1-bearing T lymphocytes in peripheral blood. It remains to be elucidated whether this finding reflects a relevant factor in the aetiology or pathogenesis of Crohn's disease.

References

1. McDermott, R.P. and Stenson, W.F. (1988). Alterations of the immune system in ulcerative colitis and Crohn's disease. *Adv. Immunol.*, **42**, 285–328
2. Selby, W.S. and Jewell, D.P. (1983). T lymphocyte subsets in inflammatory bowel disease: peripheral blood. *Gut*, **24**, 99–105
3. Yuan, S.Z., Hanauer, S.B., Kluskens, L.F. and Kraft, S.C. (1983). Circulating lymphocyte subpopulations in Crohn's disease. *Gastroenterology*, **85**, 1313–1318
4. Allison, J.P. and Lanier, L.L. (1987). Structure, function, and serology of the T-cell antigen receptor complex. *Ann. Rev. Immunol.*, **5**, 503–540
5. Brenner, M.B., Strominger, J.L. and Krangel, M.S. (1988). The τδ T cell receptor. *Adv. Immunol.*, **43**, 133–192
6. Band, H., Hochstenbach, F., McLean, J., Hata, S., Krangel, M.S. and Brenner, M.B. (1987). Immunochemical proof that a novel rearranging gene encodes the cell receptor δ subset. *Science*, **238**, 682–684
7. Lanier, L.L., Ruitenberg, J.J., Allison, J.P. and Weiss, A. (1987). Biochemical and flow cytometric analysis of CD3 and Ti expression on normal and malignant T-cells. In McMichael, A.J. (ed.) *Leucocyte Typing III.*, pp. 175–178. (Oxford: Oxford University Press).
8. Bender, S.W., Kirchmann, H. and Posselt, H.G. (1986). Morbus Crohn im Kindesalter. *Wien. Klin. Wschr.*, **16**, 520–527
9. Harms, H.K., Blomer, R., Bertels-Harms, R.M., Spaeth, A. and Koenig, M. (1987). 'Paediatric Crohn's Disease Study Group'. Verlaufsbeobachtungen an Patienten mit Morbus Crohn mit Hilfe eines neu entwickelten Crohn-Aktivitäts-Indexes (PDCAI). *Monatschr. Kinderheilk.*, **137**, 566
10. Elson, C.O., James, S.P., Graeff, A.S., Berendson, R.A. and Strober, W. (1984). Hypogammaglobulinaemia due to abnormal suppressor T-cell activity in Crohn's disease. *Gastroenterology*, **86**, 569–576
11. Goodman, T. and Lefrancois, L. (1988). Expression of γδ T-cell receptor on intestinal CD8+ intraepithelial lymphocytes. *Nature (London)*, **333**, 855–858

7
Medical treatment of chronic inflammatory bowel disease

H.K. HARMS

Medical treatment of chronic idiopathic inflammatory bowel disease (IBD) implies a particular burden to the paediatrician. He has to care for life-long disease with a tendency to frequent relapses and with no curative drugs available. Repeatedly, he must decide whether a change to another drug will hopefully ameliorate the general condition of the patient or whether a surgical procedure may be preferable. In such conflicting situations he will remember the goals of conservative treatment of IBD, which include: (1) long-term suppression of inflammation; (2) recovery and maintenance of normal growth; (3) replacement of selective deficiencies; and (4) prevention of intestinal resections as long as justifiable.

Since, in the paediatric age group, well-controlled medical treatment studies are lacking, paediatricians depend on studies in adults (NCCDS and ECCDS)[1,2] although the results may not be fully transferable to the growing child. This is especially true for prednisone, the most effective anti-inflammatory drug in ulcerative colitis (UC) as well as in Crohn's disease (CD), with its catabolic and growth-inhibiting side-effects. The initial dose of 1–2 mg/kg in the acute phase with a maximum of 60 mg/day should be continued for 6–8 weeks, followed by gradual reduction to 10–15 mg and, if possible, an alternate-day therapy, which, in our experience, frequently does not prevent recurrences.

Sulphasalazine is probably the medication most frequently used to treat UC as well as CD in childhood and adolescence. It is split into 5-ASA and sulphapyridine by the colonic microflora. The liberated sulphapyridine is largely absorbed, fast or slowly acetylated in the liver and excreted in the urine as further metabolites. Although it has been shown that 5-ASA is the active anti-inflammatory agent[3,4], sulphapyridine seems to alter the bacterial

Abbreviations: P = prednisone; A = azathioprine; SASP = sulphasalazine; 5-ASA = 5-amino-salicylic acid; M = metronidazole; Hb = haemoglobin; CVC = central venous catheter; Lop = loperamide; E = semielemental diet; Zn= zinc; PCDAI = Paediatric Crohn's Disease Activity Index

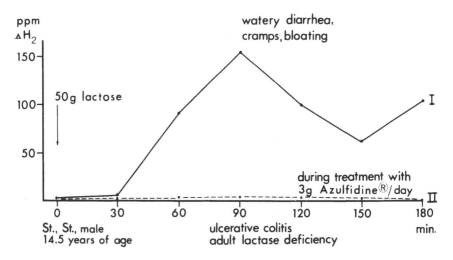

Figure 1 The effect of sulphasalazine (Azulfidine) on the H_2 producing capacity of the colonic microflora in a 14-year-old boy with adult lactase deficiency (lactase activity 4 IU) and ulcerative colitis

flora considerably[5,6]. The hydrogen breath tests in a lactose-intolerant boy with ulcerative colitis may underline this statement (Figure 1). Before treatment with sulphasalazine, he expired large amounts of hydrogen after a lactose load and nothing during treatment with Azulfidine®. Therefore, we believe that it is too early to degrade sulphapyridine as a simple carrier with considerable side reactions, especially in Crohn's disease, where the bacterial participation in the inflammatory process may be greater than in ulcerative colitis and where the effectiveness of oral 5-ASA preparations is still a matter of debate[7] and not as convincing as in ulcerative colitis. Thus, the antibacterial effect of sulphapyridine may be of some importance.

Side-effects of sulphasalazine, evaluated prospectively in the NCCDS[8], were observed in 14% of patients. But nausea, vomiting and loss of appetite, the predominant symptoms, seemed to be very unspecific as they appeared as frequently in the placebo group as in patients.

During the past 10 years, increasing interest has focused on new 5-ASA preparations. The oral preparations of mesalazine, the generic name of 5-ASA, differ in coating, pH of drug release, dose and urinary recovery (Table 1). We should be aware that the urinary excretion of oral 5-ASA products is higher than from sulphasalazine, diazosalicylate and rectally applied preparations. This elevates the potential nephrotoxicity as 5-ASA has chemical similarities to phenacetine.

Meanwhile, several convincing studies on the efficacy of oral mesalazine preparations in adult ulcerative colitis exist[9,10]. In left-sided colitis, mesalazine enemas of 4 g are as effective as local hydrocortisone[11-14]. Therefore, paediatricians should be encouraged to apply mesalazine instead of sulphasalazine in ulcerative colitis, in particular since it has become clear that oligospermia is due to the sulphapyridine moiety in sulphasalazine therapy[15].

Table 1 A selection of new orally or rectally applicable salicylate preparations

Product	Preparation	Dose	Urinary recovery
Oral			
5-ASA			
Pentasa	Mesalazine, ethyl-cellulose	250 mg	30–55%
Asacol	Mesalazine, Eudragit-S	400 mg	20–35%
Claversal, Salofalk	Mesalazine in Na/glycerin, Eudragit-S	250–500 mg	25–45%
ROW-ASA	I:Mesalazine, Eudragit	250–500 mg	60%
	II: Mesalazine, special enteric coat	250–500 mg	30%
4-ASA	Eudragit	500 mg	?
Azodisalicylate			
Dipentum	Olsalazine	250 mg	25%
Rectal			
ROW-ASA, Salofalk, Claversal	Enema pH 4.5	4 g/60 ml	
	Suppository	0.5 g/1 g	
Pentasa	Enema pH 4.8	1.2.4 g/100 ml	
4-ASA	Enema	2 g	

However, 5-ASA is also not free from side-effects[16]. They appear in 11% of patients. Skin rashes with high fever may occur, as in one of our Crohn patients. These adverse reactions had already emerged under sulphasalazine therapy and could be attributed to 5-ASA when it was given separately later on (Figure 8).

Only in CD, but not in CU, does metronidazole have an anti-inflammatory effect, especially if there is extended Crohn's colitis, fistulae and perianal involvement[17-19]. The side-effects are mainly of neurological origin and are occasionally seen in children and adolescents[20]. The potential mutagenic effect, demonstrated in animals[21], may reduce its suitability for children.

Azathioprine has no proven effect in the acute phase of IBD but is valuable in patients who require large maintenance doses of corticosteriods to remain clinically well [22-24]. It permits a significant reduction or omission of steriods but needs up to 3 months to become efficient. The necessary dose should depress the leukocyte count moderately. One third of our patients with Crohn's disease are on azathioprine.

Concerning the potential side-effects of azathioprine, the Paediatric Crohn's Disease Study Group conducted an inquiry (Table 2). Although side-effects have been reported in 26%, most of them could not be attributed to azathioprine with the exception of 7% of patients with pancreatitis. The frequency is similar to those in adults[8]. The elevated enzymes normalized rapidly after cessation of medication.

After recapitulation of the therapeutic tools for medical treatment of IBD, some special therapeutic aspects of UC and CD should be considered.

Table 2 Complications of azathioprine in 26 of 99 patients (26%) with Crohn's disease

Dermatosis (pyoderma gangrenosum 3, urticaria 1, haemorrhage 1)	8%
Pancreatitis	7%
Stenosis	5%
Abscess	3%
Sepsis, loss of hair, hypothyreote struma	3 × 1%

Results of an inquiry of the Paediatric Crohn's Disease Study Group (unpublished).

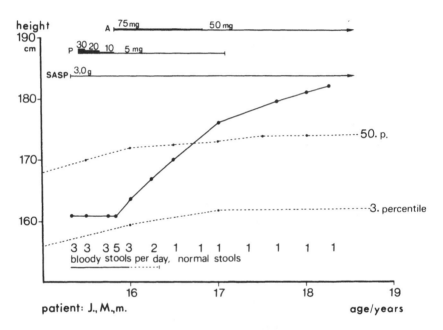

Figure 2 Male patient with ulcerative colitis and growth retardation under prednisone therapy and catch-up growth under azathioprine

In 50% of 32 patients in our department with ulcerative colitis, the inflammation was extended to the entire colon. These patients almost always needed prednisone in the acute phase of the disease. Most of them remained steroid dependent. We, therefore, add azathioprine early in order to avoid long-term growth retardation (Figure 2).

The example in Figure 3 is an 11-year-old girl with pancolitis who was initially treated in another hospital with high steroid doses and who developed severe pseudo-cushing with secondary diabetes. She was sent to us for colectomy but we first tried a combination of mesalazine and azathioprine. This therapeutic regimen resulted in normalization of height and colonic mucosa.

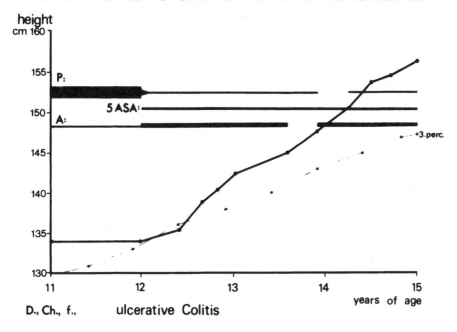

Figure 3 Female patient with ulcerative colitis and secondary diabetes recovering under the combined therapy of azathioprine with 5-ASA

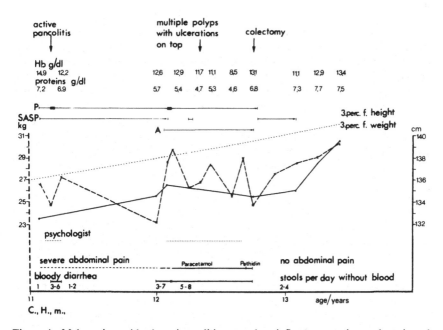

Figure 4 Male patient with ulcerative colitis, secondary inflammatory giant polyposis and unsuccessful conservative treatment

91

Table 3 Semi-elemental diet (mean 97 kcal kg^{-1} day^{-1}) and salazopryrin in the initial treatment of Crohn's disease

	Initially	After 5½ weeks of treatment	Improvement n/x patients
Weight (kg)	30.6	35.1	7/7
BSR (mm/h)	45.0	11.0	7/7
Hb (g/dl)	9.8	11.0	5/6
Leukocytes × 1000	10.24	7.8	5/7
Bands (%)	16.0	3.7	7/7
Albumin (g/dl)	2.8	3.6	7/7
α $_2$-Globulins (g/dl)	1.0	0.7	6/7
IgA (mg/dl)	313.5	199.0	7/7

The only patient who had to be colectomized was a Turkish boy in whom all our medical treatment had failed (Figure 4). On high doses of steroids, sulphasalazine and azathioprine, he continued with blood-containing diarrhoea and severe abdominal pain. Haemoglobin and proteins declined. A psychologist could not help him and the patient needed more and more analgesia. Finally, we performed colonoscopy and found multiple polyps with ulcerations on top and a normal mucosa in between. Colectomy was curative. This inflammatory pseudopolyposis is thought to occur in 20% of adult patients with long-standing UC, but is rarely seen in children[25].

Today, we recommend 5-ASA suppositories for procto-sigmoiditis and 5-ASA enemas for left-side and subtotal colitis. In the very acute phase and during remission, oral preparations may be preferable.

Since Crohn's disease is a chronic potentially life-long illness of unknown origin with high morbidity, the physician's role is to establish a sound relationship with patient and parents, and to provide information concerning the incurability of the disease and the possibilities of symptomatic and surgical therapy with an optimistic outlook. The severity of the disease depends on the localization of the disease and the time interval between first symptoms and diagnosis. At diagnosis, most children are malnourished and growth retarded, one third beyond the third percentile. Since the convincing studies of Dr Kirschner and others[26-32], we nearly always start our medical treatment in combination with semi-elemental diet. Table 3 shows that all 7 patients improved in weight and nearly all in their laboratory values. In our group, parenteral nutrition is very rare today.

Our most spectacular patient profiting from a semi-elemental diet was an 18-year-old young man without any sexual maturation and severe growth retardation (Figure 5). His height was on the 50th percentile for a 12-year-old boy. He was lost from our clinic for 6½ years on account of severe complications during parenteral nutrition at the age of eleven. In the meantime, he was under the care of a healer. Under an exclusive semi-elemental diet with 3750 kcal/day for a period of 2 years, he grew to the 3rd percentile for height and gained full sexual maturation.

About 20% of our patients with CD grow well and are without problems on sulphasalazine only. This group does not seem to be predictable. The patient in Figure 6 had extensive ileocolitis with perianal abscess which has

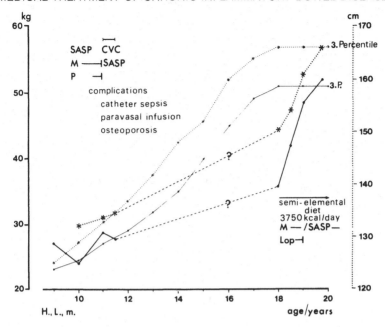

Figure 5 The effect of a two years exclusive semi-elemental diet on height and weight in a 18-year-old male patient with severe Crohn's colitis

been drained. She was considerably underweight before starting therapy and recovered rapidly without additional semi-elemental diet.

Most patients have a smouldering disease which can be controlled medically, but acute exacerbations occur from time to time and cannot be predicted or prevented. The female patient in Figure 7 is such an example. She had extensive ileocolitis up to the midcolon and suffered from severe monoarthritis of the right knee. Sulphasalazine and steroids were not helpful. With metronidazole and azathioprine she came into remission. After interruption of therapy, she suffered a full relapse. A second trial with metronidazole in combination with sulphasalazine was unsuccessful; monoarthritis reappeared. Concerning treatment with metronidazole, we learned that this drug may be effective when given the first time but not in repeated treatment. During the following 2 years, we had difficulty in controlling the disease. At age 18, the affected small intestine and colon was resected and the patient did well in the following years. This course of disease induced the speculative question of whether an earlier surgical intervention would have been more beneficial to the patient than many difficult years on partly unsuccessful medical treatment.

The difficulties in medical treatment of many patients with Crohn's disease, the high individuality of the course of the disease and the uncertainty about the best treatment, gave rise to the development of disease activity indices. The well-known Best Index[33] and van Hees Index[34] are not suitable for use in the paediatric age group since growth is not taken into consideration and clinical and laboratory variables are not well balanced.

Therefore, the Paediatric Crohn's Disease Study Group developed their

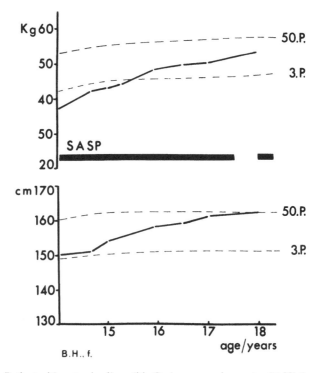

Figure 6   Patient with extensive ileocolitis Crohn, recovering under SASP therapy only

own paediatric Crohn's disease activity index (PCDAI) using stepwise regression analysis. The PCDAI is composed of the two clinical variables, appetite and number of stools/week, and four simple laboratory parameters, namely the erythrocyte sedimentation rate, serum iron, α_2-globulins and bands (Table 4).

An index score below 150 points is associated with a low disease activity, 150–220 points with a moderate and more than 220 with a high activity. In addition, we recognized the well-known clinical experience that weight changes reflect the clinical state very well. When the clinical score improved, the weight increased; when it deteriorated, there was weight loss, and when the clinical situation did not change, there was also no change in weight. As a dynamic variable, weight change could not be incorporated into the index but showed good correlation with the PCDAI. Whenever the weight decreased, the PCDAI increased and vice versa. The weight curve seems to be mirrored by the PCDAI curve.

Figure 8 shows the relationship between PCDAI and weight in an 8-year-old child. Initially, metronidazole was successful but, again, had no effect during the second period of treatment. After 3 years of therapeutic trials, the child developed zinc deficiency which was corrected by oral substitution with zinc orotrat. This seemed necessary since zinc deficiency may be a serious complication of Crohn's disease.

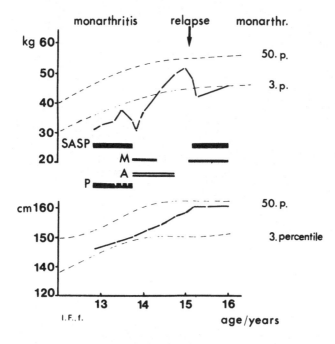

Figure 7 Example of successful combined azathioprine/metronidazole therapy and unsuccessful combination of SASP with prednisone or metronidazole in ileocolitis Crohn

Table 4 Paediatric Crohn's Disease Activity Index (PCDAI) for children and adolescents

Index = 49.7 (coefficient)	
	+ 20.2 × appetite (1,2,3)*
	+ 2.4 × stools/week
	+ 0.8 × BSR (mm/h]
	+ 4.1 × α_2-globulin (%)
	+ 1.3 × bands (%)
	− 0.3 × iron (μg/dl)

* 1 = good, 2 = moderate, 3 = severe

PCDAI range (100–350 points)

Disease activity:	Points
Low	<150
Moderate	150–220
Severe	>220

In order to test the value of regular PCDAI registrations, we compared the PCDAI of patients on conservative treatment only with the PCDAI of patients who underwent a surgical procedure. Interestingly, the PCDAIs of the two groups were significantly different with significantly higher mean

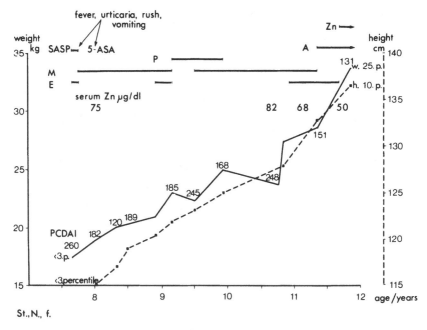

Figure 8 Female patient with Crohn's disease and the course of weight and PCDAI under changing therapy. This child showed adverse reactions to SASP and 5-ASA

PCDAI values in the group before the surgical intervention. After surgery, the PCDAI declined and adapted to the exclusively conservative-treated group during the following 3 years. This result may be interpreted as a reduction of the inflammatory mass by surgery. Further studies may help to differentiate sooner those patients who will profit from a surgical procedure.

Finally, we want to propose a flow sheet for conservative treatment of Crohn's disease in the paediatric and adolescent age groups, which we try to apply to our patients (Figure 9). We start with semi-elemental diet in combination with sulphasalazine. If a relapse occurs on sulphasalazine only, we switch to prednisone in small bowel disease, ilecolitis and severe extraintestinal manifestations, and to metronidazole in extensive Crohn's colitis, fistula and perianal disease. If these drugs are unsuccessful, the third step is azathioprine. Nutritional support should be given whenever needed.

After 1–2 years on unsuccessful conservative treatment, surgery should be considered. We believe that the development of the disease, including the therapeutic decisions, could be well monitored by the regular calculation of the paediatric Crohn's disease activity index.

References

1. Summers, R.W., Switz, D.M., Sessions, J.T. Jr., *et al.* (1979). National Cooperative Crohn's Disease Study: results of drug treatment. *Gastroenterology*, **77**, 847–869.
2. Malchow, H., Ewe, K., Brandes, J.W., Goebell, H., Ehms, H., Sommer, H. and Jesdinsky,

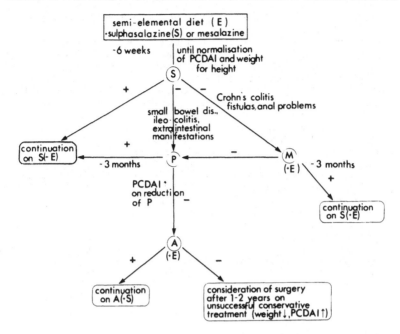

Figure 9 Flow sheet for conservative treatment of Crohn's disease in the paediatric and adolescent age groups

H. (1984). European Cooperative Crohn's Disease Study (ECCDS): results of drug treatment. *Gastroenterology*, **86**, 249–266

3. Azad Khan, A.H., Piris, J. and Truelove, S.C. (1977). An experiment to determine the active moiety of sulphasalazine. *Lancet*, **2**, 892–895
4. Klotz, U., Maier, K., Fishcher, C. and Heinkel, K. (1980). Therapeutic efficacy of sulfasalazine and its metabolites in patients with ulcerative colitis and Crohn's disease. *N. Engl. J. Med.*, **303**, 1499–1502
5. West, B., Landrun, R., Hill, M.H. and Walker G. (1974). Effects of sulphasalazine (Salazopyrin) on faecal flora. *Gut*, **15**, 960–965
6. Krook, A., Danielsson, D., Kjellander, J. and Järnerot, G. (1981). The effect of metronidazole and sulfasalazine on fecal flora in patients with Crohn's disease. *Scand. J. Gastroenterol.*, **16**, 183–192
7. Jenss, H., Hartmann F., Schölmerich, J. and the German ASA-Study Group (1989). 5-Aminosalicylic acid versus methylprednisolone in the treatment of active Crohn's disease – first results of a double blind clinical trial. *Scand. J. Gastroenterol.*, **24** (Suppl.158), 136
8. Singleton, J.W., Law, D.H., Kelley, M.L., Mekhjian, H.S. and Sturdevant, R.A.C. (1979). National Cooperative Crohn's Disease Study: Adverse reactions to study drugs. *Gastroenterology*, **71**, 870–882
9. Dew, J.W., Harries, A.D., Evans, B.K. and Rhodes, J. (1983). Treatment of ulcerative colitis with oral 5 amino salicylic acid in patients unable to take sulphasalazine. *Lancet*, **2**, 801
10. Mulder, C.J.J., Tytgat, G.N.J., Weterman, J.T., Dekker, W., Blok, P., Schrijver, M. and v.d. Heide, H. (1988). Double-blind comparison and slow-release 5-aminosalicylate and sulfasalazine in remission maintenance in ulcerative colitis. *Gastroenterology*, **95**, 1449–1453
11. Willoughby, C.P., Campieri, M., Lanfranchi, G., Truelove, S.C. and Jewell, D.P. (1986). 5-Aminosalicylic acid (Pentasa) in enema form for the treatment of active ulcerative colitis. *Ital. J. Gastroenterol.*, **18**, 15–17
12. Sutherland, L.R., Martin, F., Greer, S., Robinson, M., Greenberger, N., Saibil, F., Martin, Th., Sparr, J., Prokipchuk, E. and Borgen, L. (1987). 5-Aminosalicylic acid enema

in the treatment of distal ulcerative colitis, proctosigmoiditis, and proctitis. *Gastroenterology*, **92**, 1894-1898
13. Campieri, M., Gionchetti, P., Belluzzi, A., Tabaneli, G.M., Brignola, C., Migaldi, M., Miglioli, M. and Barbara, L. (1988). Topical treatment with 5-aminosalicylic acid as rectal enemas. In Goebell, H., Perker, B.M.V and Malchow, H. (Eds.) *Inflammatory Bowel Diseases*, pp. 357-362 (Lancaster: MTP Press Limited)
14. Biddle, W.L., Greenberger, J., Swan, T.J., McPhees, M.S. and Miner, P.B., Jr. (1988). 5 Aminosalicylic acid enemas: effective agent in maintaining remission in left-sided ulcerative colitis. *Gastroenterology*, **94**, 1075-1079
15. Rasmussen, S.N., Christensen, L., Klergaard, N., Hansen, S.H. and Lauritsen, J.G. (1989). Compromised SASP induced human sperm motility and penetration reversed with 5-ASA (Pentasa). (abstr.) *Scand. J. Gastroenterol.*, **24** (Suppl. 158), 137
16. Potvin, P.H., Peters, O., Buydens, P., Reynaert, H., Charels, K., Dehou, M.F. and Devis, G. (1989). Side effects of new 5-ASA-preparations: alopecia diffusa, reactive polyadenopathy and granulomatous hepatitis. *Scand. J. Gastroenterol.*, **24** (Suppl. 158), 140
17. Ursing, B., Alm, T., Barany, F., Bergelin, J., Gaurot-Norlin, K., Hoevels, J., Huitfeldt, B., Järnerot, G., Krause, U., Krook, A., Lindström, B., Nordle, Ö. and Rosen, A. (1982). A comparative study of metronidazole and sulfasalazine for active Crohn's disease. The cooperative Crohn's disease study in Sweden, II. Result. *Gastroenterology*, **83**, 550-562
18. Bernstein, L.H., Frank, M.S., Brandt, L.J. and Boley, S.J. (1980). Healing of perineal Crohn's disease with metronidazole. *Gastroenterology*, **79**, 357-365
19. Brandt, L.J., Bernstein, L.H., Boley, S.J. and Frank, S.S. (1982). Metronidazole therapy for perineal Crohn's disease: a follow-up study. *Gastroenterology*, **83**, 383-387
20. Duffy, L.J., Daum, F., Fisher, S.E., Selman, J., Vishnubhakat, S.M., Aiges, H.W., Markowitz, J.F. and Silverberg, M. (1985). Peripheral neuropathy in Crohn's disease patients treated with metronidazole. *Gastroenterology*, **88**, 681-684
21. Riemann, J.F. (1989). Therapie des M. Crohn. *Dtsch. Med. Wschr.*, **114**, 1620-1622
22. Present, D.H., Korelitz, B.J., Wisch, N., Glass, J.L., Sachar, D.B. and Pasternack, B.S. (1980). Treatment of Crohn's disease with 6-mercaptopurine. *N. Engl. J. Med.*, **302**, 981-989
23. O'Donoghue, D.P., Dawson, A.M., Powell-Tuck, J. *et al.* (1978). Double blind withdrawal trial of azathioprine as maintenance treatment of Crohn's disease. *Lancet*, **2**, 955-957
24. Kirk, A.P. and Lennard-Jones, J.E. (1982). Controlled trial of azathioprine in chronic ulcerative colitis. *Br. Med. J.*, **284**, 1291-1292
25. Adelson, J.W., deChadarevian, J.-P., Azouz, E.M. and Guttman, F.M. (1988). Giant inflammatory polyposis causing partial obstruction and pain in 'healed' ulcerative colitis in an adolescent. *J. Pediatr. Gastroenterol. Nutr.*, **7**, 135-140
26. Kelts, D.G., Grand, R.J., Shen, G, Watkins, J.B., Werlin, S.L. and Boehme C. (1979) Nutritional basis of growth failure in children and adolescents with Crohn's disease. *Gastroenterology*, **76**, 720-727
27. Morin, C.L., Roulet, M., Roy, C.C. *et al.* (1980). Continuous elemental enteral alimentation in children with Crohn's disease and growth failure. *Gastroenterology*, **79**, 1205-1210
28. Kirschner, B.S., Kilch, J.R., Kalman, S.S., deFavaro, M.V. and Rosenberg, I.H. (1981). Reversal of growth retardation in Crohn's disease with therapy emphasizing oral nutritional restitution. *Gastroenterology*, **80**, 10-15
29. O'Morain, C., Segal, A.M., Levi, A.J. and Valman, H.B. (1983). Elemental diet in acute Crohn's disease. *Arch. Dis. Child.*, **53**, 44-47
30. Belli, D.C., Seidman, E., Bouthillier, L. *et al.* (1988). Chronic intermittent elemental diet improves growth failure in children with Crohn's diasease. *Gastroenterology*, **94**, 603-610.
31. Aiges, H., Markowitz, J., Rosa, J. and Daum, F. (1989). Home nocturnal supplemental nasogastric feedings in growth-retarded adolescents with Crohn's disease. *Gastroenterology*, **97**, 905-910.
32. Kleinmann, R.E., Balistreri, W.F., Heyman, M.B., Kirscher, B.S., Lake, A.M., Motil, K.J., Seidman, E. and Udall, J.N. (1989). Nutritional support for pediatric patients with inflammatory bowel disease. *J. Pediatr. Gastroenterol. Nutr.*, **8**, 8-12
33. Best, W.R., Becktel, J.M., Singleton, J.W. and Kern, F. (1976). Development of a Crohn's disease activity index. *Gastroenterology*, **70**, 439-444
34. van Hees, P.A.M., van Elteren, Ph., van Lier, H.J.J. and van Tongeren, J.H.M. (1980). An index of inflammatory activity in patients with Crohn's disease. *Gut*, **21**, 279-286

8
Toxic effect of sulphasalazine on prepubertal testes

F. HADZISELIMOVIC, B. KELLER, U. HENNES and U. SCHAUB

INTRODUCTION

For almost 50 years, sulphasalazine has been the established treatment of choice for ulcerative colitis[1]. It has also been used with success in Crohn's disease, particularly when the disease involved the colon. Male infertility was recognized as a complication after prolonged sulphasalazine treatment twenty years ago[2,3].

In recent years, a growing body of evidence has been published describing the antifertility effect of Sulfosalazopyrine (SASP) both in men and rats[4-7]. The mechanism by which SASP induced seminal abnormalities remains obscure[8].

During puberty, the testes mature and sperm production starts. During this period, the testis may be particularly vulnerable to toxic influences. Both Crohn's disease and ulcerative colitis can begin prepubertally or, more commonly, at the commencement of puberty. Only preliminary results concerning the influence of SASP given chronically during the prepubertal period have been reported[9]. It seems, however, that SASP induces sterility in male rats given prepubertally[9].

The behaviour of the hypothalamo–pituitary–testicular axis in male rats treated chronically with high SASP doses per os during prepubertal as well as pubertal periods is discussed in this paper. Furthermore, the fertility rate immediately after drug discontinuation and 5 weeks after recovery is reported.

ANIMALS AND METHODS

Twenty-four male rats, 21 days old, were randomly divided into two groups of 12 animals each. One group served as control while the other group received daily 600 mg/kg sulphosalazine per os. The rats were housed separately and had the treatment for the entire period of 10 weeks. After 10 weeks, the rats were mated with 10-week-old females for one week, following which 6 rats from each group were decapitated under general anaesthesia while the remaining SASP-treated rats had a recovery period of 5 weeks. At the end of this period of time, the rats were housed again with different females, also 10 weeks old, for a period of 7 days. During the entire time, the rats had a weekly check-up (weight and general well-being) and the number as well as the weight of the newborn litters for each group was determined and compared with the controls. After decapitation, the serum was analysed for LH, FSH and testosterone determination, centrifuged and the plasma was frozen until analysed with RIA. The analysed testes were removed, weighed, and two biopsies were taken. One was fixed, in 3% glutaralaldehyde with PBS and embedded in Epon[10], semi- and ultrathin testicular sections were obtained and analysed. The second biopsies were weighed, homogenized and frozen until assayed to determine the intratesticular testosterone level. The total testicular testosterone levels were compared with those of the controls as well as with the plasma testosterone levels. Statistical analysis consisted of the Fisher exact test, Wilcoxon–Mann–Whitney U test and Spearman correlation test.

RESULTS

There was no significant difference between the body weights of the SASP-treated compared with the control rats. Both groups followed the 95th weight percentile for the entire period (Figure 1). During the first week, SASP intake was lower than 300 mg/kg body weight. But after this period, the average SASP intake was always higher than 450 mg/kg body weight (ranging from 470 to 590 mg/kg body weight) (Figure 1).

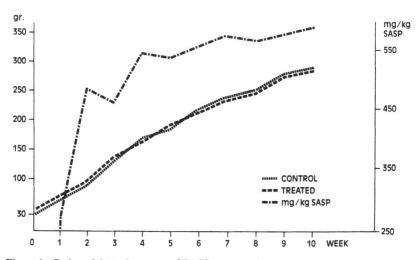

Figure 1   Body weight and amount of SASP consumed

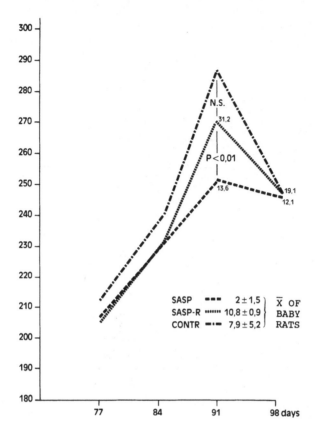

Figure 2 Significantly lower body weight was observed in pregnant female rats which had been mated with SASP-treated males. No differences in weight and number of newborns were found between the SASP recovery (SASP-R) group and controls

Females, 11 weeks old, after being mated with either controls or SASP-treated rats showed similar weight increase during the first 2 weeks of pregnancy (Figure 2). However, in the third week, the controls had significantly higher body weight increases compared with those females mated with SASP-treated rats (Figure 2).

Females mated with SASP-treated rats delivered only 2 ± 1.5 pups per litter. This was a dramatic decrease ($p < 0.02$) compared with controls (Figure 2). There was no significant decrease in the fertility rate among the groups studied. However, there were significantly more female rats born in the SASP-mated group compared with the controls or females mated with SASP-recovery group, indicating a toxic effect of SASP to androspermatozoids (Figure 3). Size of the litters, body weight, and development during the first 3 weeks of life were identical for the SASP group and controls (Figure 4). After a five-week recovery period, the pregnancy rate and the size litters in SASP-treated rats was not significantly different from controls (Figures 2 and 5).

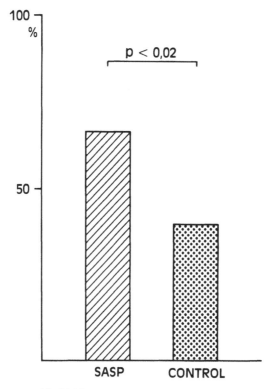

Figure 3 Treatment with SASP causes a significant adverse effect on male sperm. The ordinate represents the number of females in the litters; SASP = Sulfosalazopyrine-treated group

HISTOLOGY

The main testicular changes were observed at the late spermatids. Two distinct pathological changes were observed:

(1) Frequent nuclear degeneration, particularly prominent changes within the chromatid pattern of spermatocytes and spermatids culminating in nuclear lysis (Figures 6–8).

(2) Regularly, degenerative changes in the chromatid bodies were observed (Figures 9–12). The chromatid body appeared smaller; it was irregularly shaped and its typically electron-dense bands, as well as translucent areas, were smaller and rudimentarily developed (Figures 9–12).

Furthermore, the number of vesicles surrounding the chromatid body resembled the saccules of the Golgi apparatus and seemed to be reduced in size (Figure 10).

Degenerative changes were also observed at the level of the late spermatids (Figures 11 and 12). Bizarre nuclear shapes and peculiar perinuclear vacuoles were frequently observed. However, after 5 weeks of

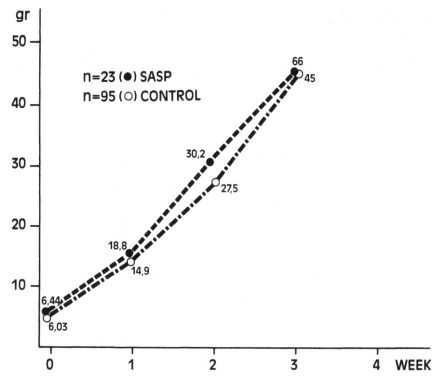

Figure 4 There is no difference in somatic development between the offspring of SASP males and that of the controls. The number at each time point represents the standard deviation. The ordinate represents the weight of each rat in grams

recovery, most of the changes described above had disappeared. No structural changes at the level of Leydig cells, Sertoli cells and spermatogonia, could be found either at light or ultrastructural level during the entire treatment period and after recovery.

Plasma LH, FSH and testosterone were identical for all three groups studied (Figures 13–15). Similarly, testicular weight and intratesticular testosterone were the same in all three groups studied (Figure 16).

DISCUSSION

The adverse effect of long-term treatment with SASP on spermatogenesis has been documented in both humans and rats[4-7,11]. However, this effect seems to be only partially reversible. Particularly, abnormal motility and pathological sperm head forms persist even months after SASP withdrawal[7]. SASP has been reported by some to produce sterility when administered to prepubertal rats[9]. However, this was not confirmed in our results, although the time when the treatment was commenced, as well as the modality of application, may be responsible for these differences. Our SASP dosages were relatively high and they were given constantly over a long period of

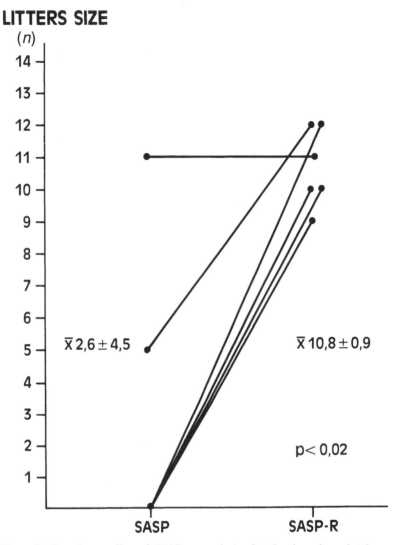

Figure 5 The adverse effect of SASP on testicular function is a time-related reversible phenomenon. Immediately after SASP-treatment, 5 out of 6 rats had a significant oligospermia which resulted in a significant decrease in the number of newborns. After a 5-week recovery period, the normal fecundity of all rats was regained

time. This has induced oligospermia due to the deleterious effects on rapidly dividing cells, particularly late spermatids. Of special interest is the observation that SASP selectively damaged more male spermatids (androspermatozoa) than female spermatids. The mechanism of this selection is as yet unknown. Pronounced nuclear as well as chromatid body changes are responsible for oligospermia, particularly since the chromatid body is known to participate at sperm axon development and therefore is responsible for the motility of sperm[12]. The permanent decrease in sperm

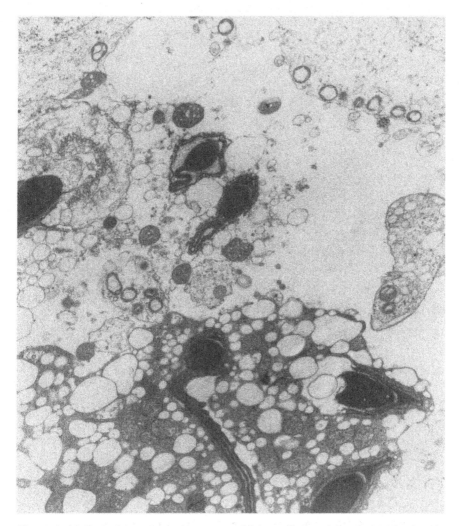

Figure 6 Malformed late spermatids were predominant findings in testicular biopsies of SASP-treated rats. ×8800

motility which has been described by others may be due to the pathological changes in the chromatid body.

Five weeks after discontinuation of SASP treatment, full recovery of fertility was achieved although some chromatid body alterations were still present. This indicates that a late but, to a great extent, completely reversible effect on spermatogenesis is initiated during puberty. The pathological changes described were not observed at the level of Leydig cells, Sertoli cells and spermatogonia. Therefore, it is not surprising that there were no hormonal changes, neither intratesticular nor in the plasma. This indicates that the pituitary–gonadal axis remained normal during the entire treatment.

105

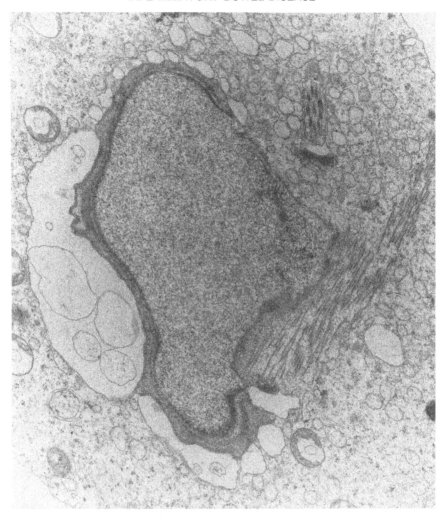

Figure 7 SASP-induced degenerative changes of spermatid-head which illustrated vacuoles and malformation of the neck of spermatid. × 20 000

Nutritional deficits have been claimed to be responsible for testicular changes in boys with leukaemia. The question remains to be answered whether SASP-induced changes together with malnutrition may have even more pronounced and lasting pathological effects at the testicular level. Therefore, a careful scrutiny for SASP treatment in males is particularly important, especially if the SASP treatment is not absolutely necessary (i.e. Crohn's disease located at caecum and terminal ileum).

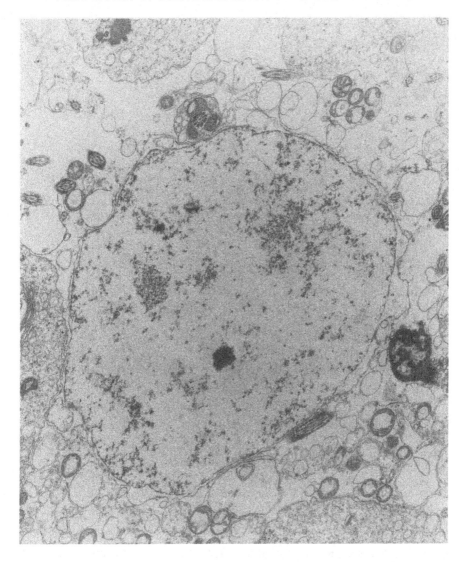

Figure 8   Nuclear-lysis often observed in SASP-treated animals. × 13 000

References

1. Svartz, N. (1942). Salazopyrin, a new sulfonilamid preparation. *Acta Med. Scand.*, **110**, 577–598
2. Fox, D.P., McKay, J.M., Brunt, P.W., Hawksworth, G.M. and Brown, J. (1987). Abnormal chromosomes and sulphasalazine therapy. In *5-ASA: The State of Art.* pp. 15–27 (Oxford, Toronto, Sydney, Philadelphia: The Medicine Publishing Foundation)
3. Toth, A. (1979). Reversible toxic effect of salicylazosulpha pyridine on semen quality. *Fertil. Steril.*, **31**, 538–540
4. Toovey, S., Hudson, E., Hendry, W.F. and Levi, A.J. (1981). Sulphasalazine and male infertility, reversibility and possible mechanism. *Gut*, **22**, 445–451
5. Birnie, G.G., McLead, T.I.F. and Watkinson, G. (1981). Incidence of sulphasalazine-

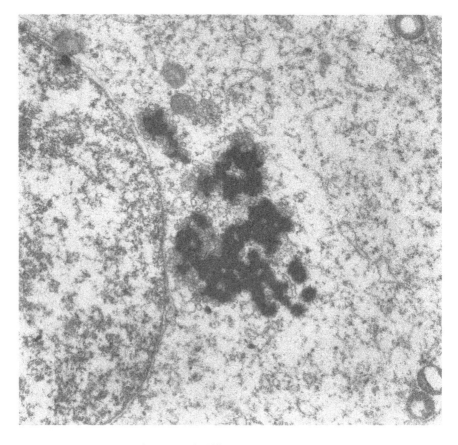

Figure 9   Normal chromatid body. × 21 000

induced male infertility. *Gut*, **22**, 452–455

6. Matus-Ridley, M., Nocosia, S.V. and Meadows, A.T. (1985). Gonadal effects of cancer therapy in boys. *Cancer*, **55**, 2353–2363
7. Riley, J.A., Lecarpentier, J., Mani, V., Goodman, M.J., Mandal, B.K. and Turnberg, L.A. (1987). Sulphasalazine induced seminal abnormalities in ulcerative colitis: results of mesalazine substitution. *Gut*, **28**, 1008–1012
8. Hrudka, F. and Singh, A. (1984). Sperm nucleomalacia in men with inflammatory bowel disease. *Arch. Androl.*, **13**, 37–57
9. Wenner, W.J., Keating, M., Piccoli, D., Watkins, J. and Levin, R. (1988). The effect of prepubertal sulphasalazine on sperm development and body weight in the rat. *Gastroenterology*, **94** (5), Part 2, 520–557
10. Hadziselimovic, F. (1977). Cryptorchidism: ultrastructure of normal and cryptorchid testis development. *Adv. Anat. Embryol. Cell Biol.*, **53**, 3
11. O'Morain, C., Smethurst, P., Dore, C.J. and Levi, A.J. (1984). Reversible male infertility due to sulphasalazine: studies in man and rat. *Gut*, **25**, 1078–1084
12. Walt, H. and Armbruster, B.L. (1984). Actin and RNA are components of the chromatoid bodies in spermatids of the rat. *Cell Tiss. Res.*, **236**, 487–490

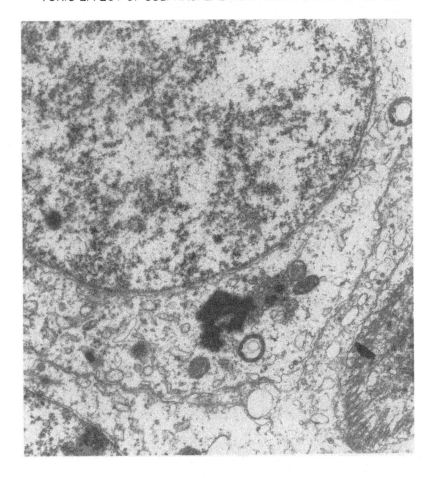

Figure 10   Pathological chromatid body of a SASP-treated rat. × 21 000

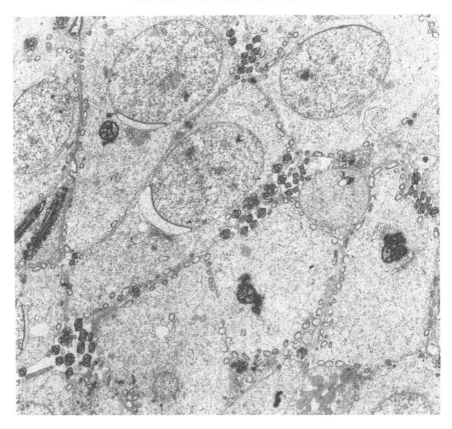

Figure 11 Electron-microscopic picture of normal spermatids which illustrates nuclear structure and chromatid bodies. × 3800

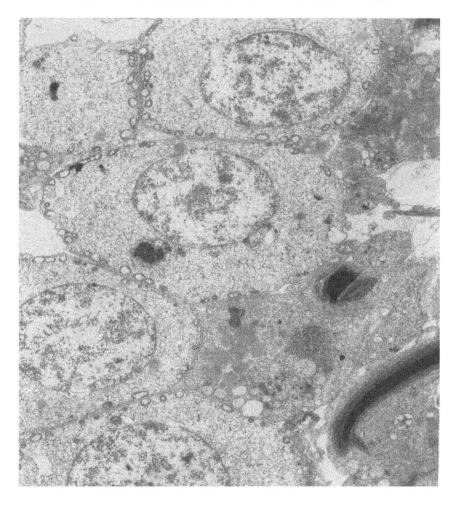

Figure 12 Pronounced pathological nuclear chromatin irregularities and degeneration of chromatid body in SASP-treated rats. × 3800

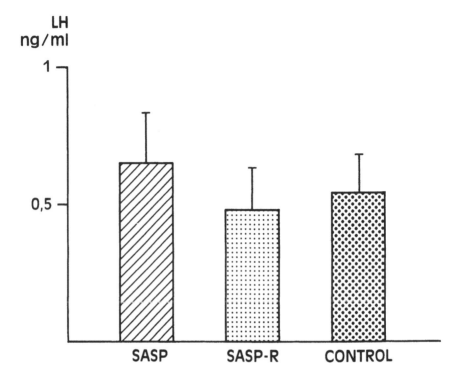

Figure 13 Normal plasma LH was found in all three groups studied. The (x) and standard deviation (SD) are represented

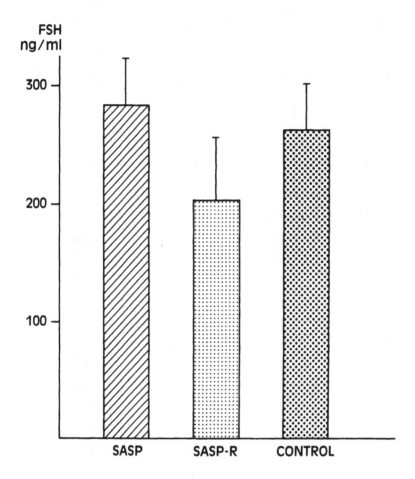

Figure 14　There was no significant difference in plasma FSH between treated and untreated rats

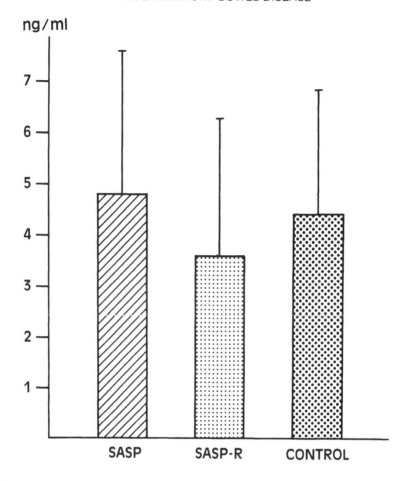

Figure 15 Normal plasma testosterone was observed in all three groups of male rats

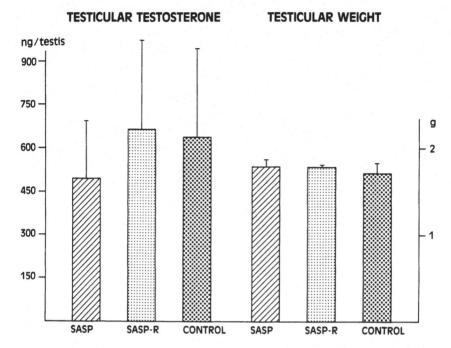

Figure 16 Testicular testosterone and testicular weight remained unchanged in all three groups studied (SASP = Salazopyrine-treated rats, SASP-R = Salazopyrine-treated rats after five weeks of recovery, and control rats)

9
Indications for surgery in inflammatory bowel disease in children

B. HERZOG

About 15–30% of inflammatory bowel disease patients are under 20 years of age (Crohn's disease about 18–30%, ulcerative colitis about 15–20%). The incidence of surgery in Crohn's disease before adulthood[1] is about 50–70%, whereas, in ulcerative colitis, it is much less[2], about 20–30%.

In paediatric patients with chronic inflammatory bowel disease, particular attention must be given to growth patterns and physical, mental and emotional development. Knowledge of pubertal changes and growth parameters is imperative in caring for paediatric patients with chronic inflammatory bowel disease.

Indications for surgical intervention in patients younger than 20 years old are consistent with indications for surgery in adult patients with the exception of growth retardation, mainly in Crohn's disease, and prevention of carcinoma in ulcerative colitis. There are absolute and relative features that indicate the need for surgery (Table 1).

PROGNOSIS OF EMERGENCY OPERATIONS FOR SEVERE COMPLICATIONS

In the group of absolute indications for surgery, free perforation, massive haemorrhage, toxic megacolon and acute fulminating colitis are life-threatening complications and medical catastrophes with high mortality and morbidity. Emergency operations for these complications are reported to have a *10–20 times higher mortality rate and a doubling of the morbidity* compared with surgical procedures done electively for inflammatory bowel disease. Therefore, whenever possible, surgery should be *elective. Earlier* operative intervention before outburst of these severe complications can result in lower mortality and morbidity.

GROWTH RETARDATION AND INDICATIONS FOR SURGERY

There is much evidence that surgery is not only helpful but necessary in children who have growth failure in Crohn's disease. In the retrospective study of Castile et al.,[1] reporting 177 children with Crohn's disease, it was significant that patients in the surgical group increased their height percentiles between the time of initial diagnosis and the final adult height in contrast to the non-surgical group in which the height percentile decreased. In addition, the surgical group at any height – whether short or tall – grew more than the patients in the non-surgical group.

If conservative treatment and a trial with total parenteral nutrition prove inadequate and active bowel disease continues in association with no measurable improvement in the rate of growth, elective surgical resection should be strongly considered. One condition has been emphasized: surgery should be planned in such a way that the anticipated postoperative remission of the disease will coincide with the pubertal growth spurt. Therefore, poor response to medical therapy in prepubertal children resulting in growth failure is an *indication* for elective surgery. The fact that simple bypass procedures cannot influence growth failure provides evidence that severely diseased bowel seems to have a direct influence on growth and sexual development[3].

In contrast, growth failure in children with ulcerative colitis is rare. But intractability and/or significant interference with quality of life because of chronic pain, Cushing appearance as a side-effect of steroids, chronic bleeding and suicidal intentions are frequent in the pre-pubertal child with ulcerative colitis. In these children, one should not hesitate to perform an elective radical and curative procedure because of its dramatic effect on the improvement of quality of life. With Telander, we would like to say that, in many ways, chronic ulcerative colitis may be considered a surgical disease[1].

Table 1 Features that characterize both ulcerative colitis and Crohn's disease

	Ulcerative colitis	Crohn's disease
Absolute features		
Massive bleeding	+++	+
Acute perforation	+++	+++
Toxic megacolon	++	++
Fistulae and abscess		
formation – intra-abdominal	+	+++
– perineal	+	+++
Acute fulminating colitis	++	+
Intestinal obstruction	(+)	+++
Relative features		
Intractability and/or		
interference with		
quality of life	+++	+++
Growth retardation	(+)	+++

RECURRENCE AND ADDITIONAL SURGERY IN CROHN'S DISEASE

Fear of recurrence after surgery may influence indications for surgery in Crohn's disease. Only 50% of paediatric patients with Crohn's disease having undergone surgical treatment will have a recurrence of the disease in 8–10 years[4]. The probability of additional surgery seems to be related to the location of the diseased bowel and number of previous operations. The presence of ileocolic disease is associated with a higher recurrence rate for surgery than other anatomic locations.

In the retrospective study of Castile et al.[1], 119 patients under 20 years of age had definitive surgery. Of these 119 patients, 96 (81%) had one or two operations whereas 23 patients (19%) had three or more definitive procedures. Evaluating these figures, with Beart et al.[5] we think that delaying operation on the basis of fear of recurrence and additional surgery is unrealistic in Crohn's disease because:

(1) Conservative resection primarily removes diseased bowel that will never return to normal,

(2) Many patients – approximately 50% – will never have recurrence of disease, and

(3) Those who have recurrence will have experienced varying periods when they were free of disease and released of the serious complications for which their operations were performed.

The value of surgery in the treatment of patients with chronic *ulcerative colitis* can be stated even more positively because recurrence of disease is never a concern after radical operation (proctocolectomy). Definite operation in ulcerative colitis is curative.

THREE REMARKS ON ANORECTAL AND PERINEAL PROBLEMS AND SURGERY

(1) When Crohn's disease of the proximal bowel responds to medical measures, the anorectal and perineal lesions usually subside as well. Surgical resections of disease in the intestine above often have similar rewards.

(2) Attempts to operate on the anorectal lesions in Crohn's disease, applying the established surgical procedures locally, usually not only fail, but also may aggravate the pre-existing conditions.

(3) Ulceration of the anal canal is a frequent finding; rectal ulcer may be the nidus of a tremendous abscess or may progress to a recto-vaginal fistula in females. Abscess is an indication for adequate incision and drainage. Penetrating anorectal ulcers are indications for aggressive surgical management.

CONCLUDING REMARKS

Indications for surgery in chronic inflammatory bowel disease in childhood should be concentrated on three preventative goals:

(1) Prevention of life-threatening complications,
(2) Prevention of growth failure and sexual underdevelopment, and
(3) Prevention of poor quality of life and emotional disturbance.

Surgery is curative in patients with chronic ulcerative colitis. It also allows intermittent relaxation in patients with Crohn's disease.

References

1. Castile, R.G., Telander, R.L., Cooney, D.R., Ilstrup, D.M., Perrault, J., van Heerden, J. and Stickler, G.B. (1980). Crohn's disease in children: assessment of the progression of disease, growth, and prognosis. *J. Pediatr. Surg.*, **15**, 462–469
2. Raine, P.A.M. (1984). BAPS collective review. Chronic inflammatory bowel disease. *J. Pediatr. Surg.*, **19**, 18–23
3. Benner, J., Weintraub, W.H., Wesley, J.R. *et al.* (1979). Crohn's disease in children and adolescents: Is inadequate weight gain a valid indication for surgery? *J. Pediatr. Surg.*, **14**, 325–328
4. Kibort, Ph.M. (1987). Inflammatory bowel disease in childhood. *J. Enterostomal Ther.*, **14**, 79–82
5. Beart, R.W. Jr. *et al.* (1980) *Surgical Management of Inflammatory Bowel Disease. Current Problems in Surgery.* (New York: Year Book)

10
Surgery for inflammatory bowel disease: ulcerative colitis

A. COLODNY

Ulcerative colitis is a diffuse inflammatory process involving primarily the mucosal layer of the rectum and the colon. The aetiology of this disease remains obscure. Medical management may be helpful in controlling the symptoms but is not curative. Surgical removal of the colon and rectum cures this disease since ulcerative colitis is limited to the colon and rectum and does not involve the small intestine. However, in the past, it was necessary to have a stoma and to wear an appliance in order to achieve this cure.

Recently, preservation of continence by one surgical technique or another has been developed. This allows surgery to be considered at an earlier stage in the disease process since the patient may find a surgical cure with preservation of faecal continence much more acceptable than surgical cure of the disease with a stoma and an appliance. A previous presentation (Professor Dr B. Herzog, Chapter 9) has clearly outlined the indications for surgery and they will not be discussed further.

HISTORICAL PERSPECTIVE

The first recorded description of the pathological features of ulcerative colitis[1] was by Samuel Wilks MD, pathologist and physician at Guy's Hospital in London. In a series of lectures on pathological anatomy, given during the summer sessions of 1857 and 1858, he described a form of colitis involving primarily the mucosa. That description would be valid today in cases that have come to be known as idiopathic ulcerative colitis. Surgical techniques for the management of a patient with ulcerative colitis were recorded at the end of the 19th century. In 1893, Mayo Robson[2] reported a case of colitis with ulceration which was treated by inguinal colotomy in order to allow instillation of ipecacuanha and hammaemelis to try to alleviate the pain, bleeding and mucous discharge that had failed to respond to the ordinary forms of medical treatment and instillations per anus. Eventually, the ulcerations healed and the faecal fistula was closed with a satisfactory result. In 1902, Robert Weir MD, who was professor of surgery at the College of Physicians and Surgeons in New York, reported the use of the appendix as a conduit to allow irrigation with a 5% solution of methyl blue alternating with a solution of nitrate of silver 1-5000 or of bismuth to attempt to cure the ulcerative process[3]. Dr Weir had actually been planning to do a caecostomy but the appendix rose so suggestively into view that he employed it to make the desired fistula.

In 1931, Dr John Young Brown[3] from St Louis proposed that complete physiological rest of the large bowel was the key to bringing about a remission in patients with ulcerative colitis and proposed the use of an end ileostomy to achieve this. He planned to close the stoma after a 'cure' had been achieved. In 1943, Sir Hugh Devine from Melbourne Australia described a multiple-staged method of partial colectomy for patients with ulcerative colitis who were in very poor condition[5]. In 1944, A.A. and A.F. Strauss[6] introduced the first successful ileostomy appliance consisting of a sheet-metal circular disc covered with rubber with a hole in the centre for the ileal stoma. A flat rubber pouch with an outlet spout at the bottom was attached to the disc for collection of the ileostomy discharge and evacuation of the same. An elastic belt was fastened to hooks on each side of the disc which was cemented to the abdomen with rubber cement. This made ileostomy a socially more acceptable procedure but there were a number of complications with the appliance, many of which were related to the fact that the cements used have a property called 'creep' in the physics of the materials. Therefore, a search for surgical techniques which would eliminate the need for appliances continued and will be discussed below.

In 1948 Richard Cattell[7] of the Lahey Clinic in Boston came to the conclusion that ileostomy without removal of the diseased colon and rectum was not beneficial and that most patients who required an ileostomy would eventually need removal of a portion or all of the colon and rectum. He described a three-stage approach consisting of end ileostomy, followed by subtotal colectomy and then, as a final stage, the abdominal perineal resection of the rectum. Because of the fact that many of the patients were referred for stomal surgery only as a last resort (frequently debilitated and sometimes moribund), it was felt that they were too sick to have resection of the colon and underwent ileostomy only. This left all the diseased colon in place with ongoing infection, toxaemia, and protein, electrolyte and blood loss. The resulting mortality was unacceptable. The concept that these patients were too sick to leave the diseased colon in place led to carrying out a partial colectomy simultaneously with the ileostomy. Thus, in 1949, Dr Gavin Miller et al.[8] from Montreal proposed accomplishing the surgical removal of all the diseased bowel in two stages. The first stage was an ileostomy and a partial colectomy down to the lower sigmoid. One could either create a sigmoid mucous fistula or a Hartmann's pouch. This resulted in a significant decrease in both mortality and morbidity. The second stage would be an abdominal perineal resection of the sigmoid and rectum. In 1951, Mark Ravitch and Handelsman[9] from the Department of Surgery at the Johns Hopkins Hospital proposed a one-stage operation consisting of an ileostomy and a total proctocolectomy. This was considered to be a major advance at that time but it did remove the rectum precluding an ileorectostomy or an ileoanal pullthrough. Some surgeons had been leaving the rectum in place for a variable period of time depending on the symptoms and the pathological condition of the rectum, hoping it would eventually prove useful. It was also a psychologic boost to a patient having a stoma created that there was some remote hope of re-establishment of faecal continence.

In 1952, a major advance was recorded by Mr Brooke[10] when he suggested maturing the ileostomy stoma at the time of surgery rather than waiting for this to be accomplished spontaneously. Prior to this report, the terminal ileum had been left protruding from the ileostomy site waiting for it to turn back on itself. This resulted in serositis and partial intestinal obstruction, with a so-called 'spitting' ileostomy with loss of large quantities of fluids and electrolytes and/or significant scarring and stricturing of the stoma. Maturing the stoma at the time it was created has virtually eliminated these complications.

PRESERVATION OF FAECAL CONTINENCE

As mentioned previously, Sir Hugh Devine[5] felt that temporizing half measures, such as appendicostomy, caecostomy, or enterostomy, were not of any permanent avail in patients with significant ulcerative colitis. He felt that nothing short of colectomy would save such a patient's life. However, in 1943, many of these patients presented for surgical treatment in a late stage of the disease with great emaciation and debility. He proposed a staged approach to establishing an ileostomy and removing the majority of the colon in these moribund patients. This included the formation of a Mikulicz spur between the terminal ileum and the sigmoid colon. After multiple stages, in which the colon was gradually removed, the spur was crushed and then the ileal sigmoid fistula was closed to re-establish continuity of the intestinal tract. The patient survived and did reasonably well with few immediate symptoms from the remaining rectum and small amount of sigmoid.

In 1947, Dr Mark Ravitch and Sabiston[11] reported a case in which a young girl with familial polyposis had an ileostomy and partial colectomy and an ileosigmoidostomy. Some eight years after the removal of the colon, she returned with an adenocarcinoma of the rectum causing obstruction and subsequently died. This occurred despite several sigmoidoscopic examinations for recurrent polyps with fulguration of any residual polyps. Because of this disaster, he suggested removal of the entire colon, resection of the mucosa of the rectum and lower sigmoid and a pullthrough of the terminal ileum with anastomosis of the ileum to the anus. He reported his results in 28 dogs and was encouraged to try it in humans in a staged approach. However, because of problems with frequent stools, fluid and electrolyte losses, infection, etc., the operation did not gain wide acceptance.

In 1903, Lilienthal[12] performed a total colectomy with an ileosigmoid anastomosis, thereby preserving the rectum and attempting to maintain faecal continence, clearly an advantage over the then current 'venting' procedures. In 1953, Stanley Aylett[13] in Great Britain and later, in 1963, Owen Wangensteen *et al.*[14] in the United States reported encouraging results in patients who had a primary ileorectostomy after removal of the colon for ulcerative colitis. Even though it was acknowledged that improvements in ileostomy appliances had relieved some of the terrors of an ileostomy, it was felt that the results obtained by Devine[5] could be achieved with a primary anastomosis and a one-stage procedure rather than a multiple-stage procedure. Aylett[15] ultimately reported 300 patients and claimed that persistent symptoms due to retention of the inflamed rectal mucosa were not significant and that the possibility of developing carcinoma in the retained diseased mucosa was not as great as had been suggested. However, many surgeons disagreed with his point of view and this procedure has not had wide acceptance. If it is carried out, periodic endoscopy must be pursued for the rest of the patient's life. This operation may enjoy a revival if the complications from the ileal–anal pullthrough become significant. This is particularly true since the incidence of developing carcinoma in the retained rectosigmoid was somewhat exaggerated initially. A monitoring system, including periodic total colonoscopy, in patients with chronic ulcerative colitis for longer than 10 years who are otherwise doing well and have not had surgery has been established hopefully to pick up premalignant epithelial dysplasia before a true carcinoma has developed. It may be argued that monitoring after an ileorectostomy would be easier than when the entire colon remains.

Meanwhile, in 1969, Kock[16] presented the initial results of a continent ileostomy which consisted of an antiperistaltic pouch with a nipple valve. While this still involved an abdominal wall stoma, the use of an appliance was not required. Despite a significant number of problems with this procedure, it still, when it worked, offered a quality of life superior to that with a conventional ileostomy.

Ileoanal anastomoses had been tried for various malignant and benign conditions after surgical removal of the rectum. Many of these early efforts of enteroanostomy after protectomy were complicated by anastomotic breakdown, pelvic abscesses and fistulae.

Mucosal stripping transanally was tried late in the 19th century and this actually resulted in a decrease in morbidity and mortality. It was Soave's demonstration[17] in 1964 of the safety of rectal mucosectomy that led to the application of this technique in the construction of the enteroanal anastomosis. After trying the ileoanal pullthrough after a mucosectomy in dogs, Mark Ravitch[18] reported success in two patients. Initial results for this complex and technically difficult and lengthy operation were discouraging because of frequent complications. However, when a proximal temporary ileostomy was added in 1951, the complication rate decreased.

The optimistic reports from Droboni[19] in 1967, Martin *et al.*[20] in 1977 and Ekesparre *et al.*[21] in 1978 of unprecedented success, despite the intricate nature of the operation, in patients who had meticulous and prolonged preoperative preparation rekindled the interest in this operative procedure.

In 1980, Parks and Nicholls[22] reported the addition of an S pouch to the procedure to try to decrease the frequency of bowel movements. In 1982, Utsunomiya et al.[22] created a J pouch as a substitute for the S pouch. The J pouch was easier to construct than the S pouch and the J pouch facilitated evacuation of the neorectum spontaneously in a greater proportion of patients than the S-shaped pouch. In addition, the fact that the pelvic dissection was performed endorectally meant that there should be very few or no complications related to neurogenic dysfunction of the bladder or the sexual apparatus of males.

SURGICAL ALTERNATIVES FOR THE PATIENT WITH ULCERATIVE COLITIS (Figure 1)

Total protocolectomy with conventional ileostomy

Although performed relatively infrequently today, this procedure still remains a benchmark. It is curative and relatively simple. It does require an abdominal wall stoma and appliance. There are a number of complications related to the abdominal perineal resection of the rectum and the posterior wound. These consist of neurogenic dysfunction of the bladder and sexual apparatus in the male, pelvic abscesses, posterior wound infections and draining sinuses. There are also some potential complications related to the ileostomy but these have been minimized since the introduction by Mr Brooke[10] of the matured stoma. Modern-day appliances have also eliminated many of the stomal and appliance problems.

Total colectomy without protectomy and ileorectal anastomosis

While this procedure does maintain faecal continence with preservation of the sphincters, it has the theoretical disadvantage of retaining some rectal mucosa which may cause persistence of the patient's symptoms and also is at risk to develop carcinoma. These theoretical disadvantages have become real as time has gone by but many have been somewhat exaggerated initially. It has found limited acceptance except in special situations where an external stoma or the potential complications of an ileoanal pullthrough would be difficult to manage. It does require rather frequent periodic endoscopy. The development of the ileoanal pullthrough with rectal mucosectomy has led to a decline in enthusiasm for the ileorectostomy.

Continent ileostomy (Kock pouch)

This procedure involves creation of an antiperistaltic pouch and a nipple valve to prevent incontinence. It does require a stoma and intermittent catheterization to empty the pouch. A number of complications with this procedure have limited its acceptance. Most of the significant complications

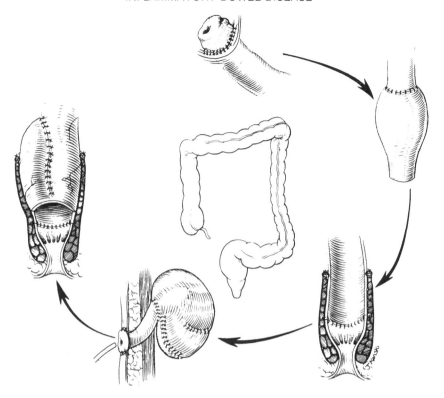

Figure 1 This figure diagrammatically illustrates the current surgical alternatives for a patient with ulcerative colitis who has failed medical management, namely: permanent ileostomy with total proctocolectomy; total colectomy with ileorectal anastomosis; Kock continent ileostomy; and ileoanal pullthrough with or without construction of a pouch

are related to the failure of the nipple valve. It does provide a suitable alternative for the patient who has had a previous protectomy or the patient who has had failure of the ileoanal pullthrough procedure but who still desires to have a continent procedure carried out.

Ileoanal pullthrough

When successful, this provides faecal continence without requiring an external appliance, stoma or intermittent catheterization. It has a number of complications (Table 1) and is a tedious, technically difficult operation to perform. Even when it works, it requires understanding and patience from patients since multiple (5–8) bowel movements a day are not uncommon.

Table 1 Ileoanal pullthrough complications

Complication	Occurrence
Daytime incontinence	1–3%
Nocturnal incontinence	5–13%
Stool frequency	5–8/day
Pelvic or cuff abscess	1–3%
Small bowel obstruction	10%
Permanent ileostomy	5%

Table 2 The advantages and disadvantages of ileostomy and proctocolectomy

Advantages	Disadvantages
Time tested	Stoma and bag
Relatively simple	Pelvic dissection
Curative	Perineal wound
	Metabolic

Table 3 The advantages and disadvantages of ileorectostomy

Advantages	Disadvantages
Simple; no stoma	Residual disease
Continence; no bag	Cancer risk
Sit to stool	Persistent symptoms
No pelvic dissection	
No perineal wound	

Table 4 The advantages and disadvantages of Kock continent ileostomy

Advantages	Disadvantages
Curative	Catheterization
No bag	Pouchitis
Frequency	Dessusception (10%)
Urgency	Reoperation (15–25%)
	Stoma

Table 5 The advantages and disadvantages of ileoanal endorectal pullthrough

Advantages	Disadvantages
Curative	Frequent bowel movements
Continence	Pouchitis
Sit to stool	Complex operation
No stoma	Salt-losing state
No bag	
No catheter	

Conclusion

Basically, at present, there are four surgical alternatives for the patient with ulcerative colitis for whom medical therapy has failed. Each of these four has certain advantages and certain disadvantages (Tables 2–5). Complete discussion of these advantages and disadvantages must be carried out with the patient and/or the family. Since those procedures which preserve faecal continence are concerned primarily with quality of life rather than restoration of health, careful consideration of all available facts must be undertaken before an intelligent choice can be made.

References

1. Wilks, S. (1859). *Lectures on Pathologic Anatomy*. (London: Longman, Brown, Green, Longmans and Roberts, Paternoster Row)
2. Robson, M. (1893). Case of colitis with ulceration treated by inguinal colotomy and local treatment of the ulcerated surfaces with subsequent closure of the artificial anus. *Trans. Clin. Soc. London,* **26**, 213
3. Weir, R.F. (1902). A new use for the useless appendix in the surgical treatment of obstinate colitis. *Med. Rec.,* **62**, 201
4. Brown, J.Y. (1923). Value of complete physiologic rest of large bowel in certain ulcerative and obstructive lesions. *Surg. Gynecol. Obstet.,* **16**, 610
5. Devine, H. (1943). A method of colectomy for desperate cases of ulcerative colitis. *Surg. Gynecol. Obstet.,* **76**, 136
6. Strauss, A.A. and Strauss, A.F. (1944). Surgical treatment of ulcerative colitis. *S. Clin. N. Am.,* **24**, 211
7. Cattell, R.B. (1948). The surgical treatment of ulcerative colitis. *Gastroenterology,* **10**, 63
8. Miller, C.G. *et al.* (1949). Primary resection of the colon in ulcerative colitis. *J. Can. Med. Assoc.,* **60**, 584
9. Ravitch, M.M. and Handelsman, J.C. (1951). One stage resection of entire colon and rectum for ulcerative colitis and polypoid adenomatosis. *Bull. Johns Hopkins,* **88**, 59
10. Brooke, B.N. (1952). The management of an ileostomy including its complications. *Lancet,* **2**, 102
11. Ravitch, M.M. and Sabiston, D.C. (1947). Anal ileostomy with preservation of the sphincter. *Surg. Gynecol. Obstet.,* **84**, 1095
12. Lilienthal, H. (1903). Extirpation of the entire colon, the upper portion of the sigmoid flexure and four inches of the ileum for hyperplastic colitis. *Ann. Surg.,* **37**, 616
13. Aylett, S.O. (1953). Conservative surgery in the treatment of ulcerative colitis. *Br. Med. J.,* **2**, 1348
14. Wangensteen, O.H., Griffen, W.O. and Lillehei, R.C. (1963). Ileo-proctostomy in ulcerative colitis. *Surgery,* **50**, 75
15. Aylett, S.O. (1966). Three hundred cases of diffuse ulcerative colitis treated by total colectomy and ileorectal anastomosis. *Br. Med. J.,* **1**, 1001
16. Kock, N.G. (1969). Intra-abdominal "reservoir" in patients with permanent ileostomy. Preliminary observations on a procedure resulting in fecal "continence" in five ileostomy patients. *Arch. Surg.,* **99**, 223
17. Soave, F. (1964). A new surgical technique for the treatment of Hirschsprung's disease. *Surgery,* **56**, 1007
18. Ravitch, M.M. (1948). Anal ileostomy with sphincter preservation in patients requiring total colectomy for benign conditions. *Surgery,* **24**, 170
19. Droboni, S. (1967). One stage proctocolectomy and anal ileostomy: Report of 35 cases. *Dis. Colon Rectum,* **10**, 143
20. Martin, L.W., LeCoultre, C. and Schubert, W.K. (1977). Total colectomy and mucosal protectomy with preservation of continence in ulcerative colitis. *Ann. Surg.,* **186**, 477

21. Ekesparre, W. and Von Janneck, C. (1978). Follow-up results of the pull-through operation for ulcerative colitis in children. In *Progress in Pediatric Surgery*, Vol. VII, pp. 7–20. (Baltimore and Munich: Urban and Schwartzenberg)

22. Parks, A.G. and Nicholls, R.J. (1978). Protocolectomy without ileostomy for ulcerative colitis. *Br. Med. J., 2*, 85

23. Utsunomiya, J., Iwama, T., Imajo, M. *et al.* (1980). Total colectomy, mucosal protectomy and ileoanal anastomosis. *Dis. Colon Rectum, 23*, 459

11
Factors that influence the postoperative recurrence of Crohn's disease in childhood

A.M. GRIFFITHS

Despite the likelihood of eventual disease recrudescence the possibility of a significant asymptomatic interval following intestinal resection in Crohn's disease makes such surgery an attractive therapeutic option. This is particularly true for children and adolescents, for whom delay in growth and pubertal development is a common and disturbing complication, and for whom the adverse effects of steroids and the inconvenience of nutritional therapies frequently become unacceptable. Rates of variably defined 'recurrence' have been documented[1-3] and influential factors have been analyzed amongst adult patients[4-6,8] but not children. Such paediatric data are necessary, as young age has been reported by some to adversely affect outcome.

We recently reviewed the postoperative outcome of young patients with Crohn's disease, surgically treated at the Hospital for Sick Children in Toronto. Recurrence was defined as both return of intestinal symptoms and radiologic demonstration of mucosal disease. Cumulative recurrence rates were calculated in order to correct for the varying lengths of follow-up. Our main aim was to identify factors which influence the length of the postoperative disease-free interval. Can one predict who is and who is not likely to gain a substantial symptom-free period during which normal growth may occur?

Patients were stratified into subgroups according to sex, anatomic location of disease, indication for operation, use of preoperative bowel rest, preoperative duration of symptomatic disease and pathologic characteristics of the resected intestine. Postoperative recurrence-free survival curves for the various subgroups were compared using Wilcoxon and log rank procedures.

Between 1970 and 1987, eighty-nine patients with Crohn's disease, out of a total of 275 followed by the Inflammatory Bowel Diseases Clinic, underwent their first intestinal resection at The Hospital for Sick Children. There was one late postoperative death due to a series of septic complications. Six patients were lost to follow-up within the first postoperative year. The remaining 82 surgically treated patients, followed for a mean of 5.3 ± 3.3 years, constitute the study group. Their mean age at the time of operation was 14.8 years (range 5.9–19.0 years). The median postoperative recurrence-free survival for the entire group was 5.1 years. The majority of patients underwent intestinal resection with primary reanastomosis. Only 5 (2 with colonic Crohn's disease and 3 with extensive ileocolonic involvement) were treated with resection and ileostomy.

Anatomic localization of disease was the most important factor influencing the length of the postoperative disease-free interval. The largest group of patients undergoing intestinal resection consisted of 46 with disease confined to the terminal ileum, with or without cecal involvement. Ten patients had more proximal and often more extensive small bowel disease, but a normal colon. Both the distal ileum and the colon were abnormal in 24 patients. Of these, colonic inflammation was limited to the right colon in 8, but was diffuse and extensive in 16. Only 2 patients had disease confined to the colon, precluding any meaningful statement about their outcome. This small number is due to our reluctance to include patients suspected of having colonic Crohn's disease, but in whom the diagnosis remained indeterminant even after pathologic examination of the resected colon.

The recurrence rates for the extensive ileocolonic disease group are strikingly different from those of all other anatomical subgroups (Figure 1) (p <0.0001). The median disease-free survival was only 1 year for patients with extensive ileocolonic disease compared with 5 years for the terminal ileal ± cecal group and 6 years for the small bowel group. The outcome of patients with disease in the terminal ileum and right (i.e. ascending) colon was similar to the ileal and small bowel groups.

The second factor influencing rate of disease recrudescence was indication for operation (Table 1). Forty-six patients were treated surgically for 1 or more intestinal complications such as bowel obstruction, intra-abdominal abscess, enterovesicular or enterocutaneous fistula, perforation or major haemorrhage. (Enteroenteric fistula was never considered an absolute indication for resection.) In 31, resection was carried out because of 'failure of medical therapy' without such a specific intestinal complication. The remaining 3 patients came to operation 'for diagnosis' prior to any medical therapy, because of concern about a radiologic appearance of malignancy in 2 and for suspected acute appendicitis in 1.

In the surgical group as a whole, patients undergoing resection for a specific intestinal complication enjoyed a longer postoperative recurrence-free interval (median of 6.0 years) than those who simply failed medical therapy (median recurrence-free survival of 1.7 years). The discrepant survival curves of patients so stratified are shown in Figure 2 (p < 0.003). This observation is partly explained by the preponderance of patients with extensive ileocolonic disease in the group undergoing surgery without a specific intestinal complication. Nevertheless even within anatomic subgroups a similar trend was observed.

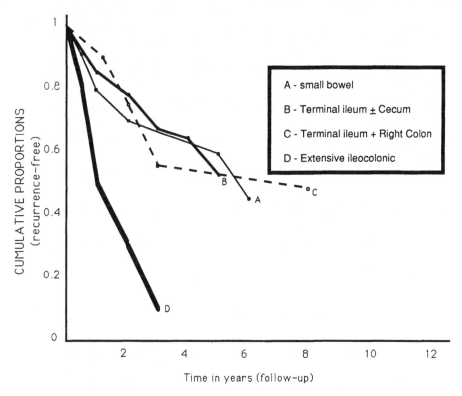

Figure 1 Cumulative postoperative recurrence-free survival according to anatomic localization of Crohn's disease

Table 1 Indications for resection (Small bowel, ileal ± cecal and ileocolonic disease)

Failure of medical therapy alone		31
Specific intestinal complication[a]		46
bowel obstruction	27	
intra-abdominal abscess	9	
enterovesicular fistula	4	
enterocutaneous fistula	7	
perforation	4	
major haemorrhage	2	
Diagnosis		3

[a] More than 1 per patient possible

Preoperative duration of symptomatic disease prior to intestinal resection was analyzed as a covariable amongst patients stratified according to anatomic localization of disease. In contrast to studies amongst adults, notably Dr David Sachar's group at the Mt Sinai Hospital in New York, we noticed a trend toward a negative correlation, i.e., shorter periods of preoperative illness were associated with more delayed recrudescence of active disease ($p < 0.05$). This same correlation reached greater statistical

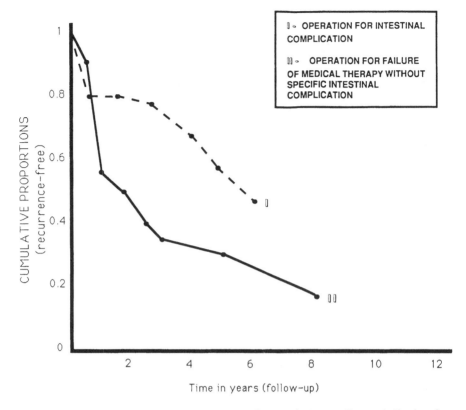

Figure 2 Cumulative postoperative recurrence-free survival according to indication for operation

significance ($p < 0.02$) amongst patients stratified according to indication for resection.

The length of the postoperative recurrence-free interval was not influenced by age, sex, use of preoperative bowel rest or presence of granulomata in the resected bowel.

Most surgery in Crohn's disease is elective. Most physicians would agree that there are many relative and a few absolute indications for operation. In choosing surgical treatment one hopes to achieve a significant disease-free interval, long enough in young patients to allow optimal growth[7]. In our patients the effect of surgery on growth was very positive.

Thirty patients were prepubertal (Tanner stage 1) or in early puberty (Tanner stage 2) at the time of intestinal resection. Their mean height velocity in the 1 year preoperatively where recorded ($n = 22$) increased in nearly all from a mean of 2.5 cm/year to a mean of 8.2 cm/year ($n = 28$) in the first postoperative year (Figure 3). Data for the 8 patients in Tanner stage 3 at the time of surgery are similar (2.2 cm/year increasing to 7.6 cm/year). Patients in Tanner stage 1, 2 or 3 ($n = 38$) increased from a mean height centile of 11.1 ± 12.6 at the time of resection to 29.5 ± ultimately ($n = 27$) or currently ($n = 11$) ($p < 0.001$).

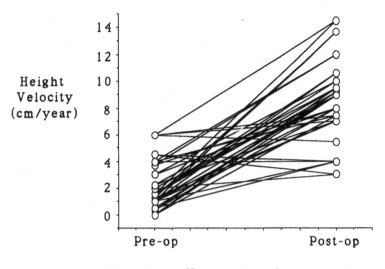

All patients Tanner 1 or 2 at resection

Figure 3 Comparison of pre- and post-operative height velocity

In summary, anatomic localization of disease was the most important factor influencing the postoperative recrudescence of Crohn's disease. Extensive ileocolonic disease was associated with a much earlier recurrence (50% by 1 year) than other subgroups (50% by 5–6 years). Patients undergoing resection for a specific intestinal complication (e.g. obstruction/abscess/perforation) experienced recurrence later than those who had simply 'failed medical therapy'. Shorter periods of preoperative disease were associated with longer postoperative recurrence-free intervals. Growth velocity improved greatly following resection in patients prepubertal or in early puberty.

Our results support early surgical management of young patients with relatively localized Crohn's disease. The excess of early recurrences in extensive ileocolonic disease suggests that for these children alternative strategies (medical or nutritional) should be sought and maintained.

References

1. Lennard-Jones, J.E. and Stalder, G.A. (1987). Prognosis after resection of chronic regional ileitis. *Gut*, **8**, 332–336
2. Greenstein, A.J., Sachar, D.B., Pasternack, B.S. and Janowitz, H.D. (1975). Reoperation and recurrence in Crohn's colitis and ileocolitis. *N. Engl. J. Med.*, **293**, 685–690
3. Hellers, G. (1979). Crohn's disease in Stockholm county 1955–74. A study of epidemiology, results of surgical treatment and long-term prognosis. *Acta Chir. Scand.*, **490** (suppl): 31–70
4. Lock, M.R., Farmer, R.G., Fazio, V.W., Jagelman, D.G.M., Lavery, I.C. and Weakley, F.L. (1981). Recurrence and reoperation for Crohn's disease. The role of disease location in prognosis. *N. Engl. J. Med.*, **304**, 1586–1588
5. Sachar D.B., Wolfson, D.M., Greenstein, A.J., Goldberg, J., Styczynski, R. and Janowitz,

H.D. (1983). Risk factors for postoperative recurrence of Crohn's disease. *Gastroenterology*, **85**, 917–921

6. Whelan, G., Farmer, R.G., Fazio, V.W. and Goormastic, M. (1985). Recurrence after surgery in Crohn's disease. Relationship to location of disease (clinical pattern) and surgical indication. *Gastroenterology*, **88**, 1826–1833.

7. Castile, R.G., Telander, R.L., Cooney, D.R., Ilstrup, D.M., Perrault, J., van Heerden, J. and Stickler, G.B. (1980). Crohn's disease in children: Assessment of the progression of disease, growth and progress. *J. Pediatr. Surg.*, **15**, 462–469

8. Greenstein, A.J., Lachman, P., Sachar, D.B., Springhorn, J., Heimann, T., Janowitz, H.D. and Aufses, A.H., Jr. (1988). Perforating and non-perforating indications for repeated operations in Crohn's disease: evidence for two clinical forms. *Gut*, **29**, 588–592

12
Psyche and inflammatory bowel disease

G. STACHER

Psychological factors have been, and in some quarters still are, held to be of significant importance for the aetiology, the timing of onset or exacerbation and the course of inflammatory bowel disease.

INTRA- AND INTERPERSONAL FACTORS

Alexander[1] thought that a specific, unconscious conflict was characteristic for patients who develop ulcerative colitis: the conflict between the wish to carry out certain obligations and to accomplish something which requires a concentrated expenditure of energy, and the unwillingness or inability to do so. The disease would break out when this conflict was activated. In such a situation, the patient would regress to the time of the first demand for accomplishment, i.e. the time of the development of bowel control, and would overcompensate the frustration of his longings by the urge to give, and substitute diarrhoea for making the required effort. The onset of the disease, however, would also necessitate a vulnerability of the involved organ on the basis of inheritance or early development.

Grace and Graham[2], as well, conceptualized inflammatory bowel disease as psychogenic. They proposed that each psychogenic illness was associated with a specific attitude expressed by the patient toward the situation that evoked the illness. This attitude contained: (a) what the person felt was happening to him; and (b) what he wished to do about it: patients with ulcerative colitis and Crohn's disease felt that they were being injured and degraded and wished they could get rid of the harmful agent.

Later, psychosomatic theorizing was not so much focused on intrapsychic conflicts but on interindividual relationships. Engel[3] reported to have found, among 39 patients with ulcerative colitis, 'with impressive consistency', not only defects in personality structure long antedating the disease onset, but also a dependent and restricted relationship with people, a consistent psychopathology in the patients' mothers, and a failure to achieve full heterosexual development. The onset and relapses had occurred in settings representing real, threatened or phantasized interruptions of key relationships, but only when the corresponding affect was helplessness, despair or hopelessness. Similarly, McDermott and Finch[4] described children with ulcerative colitis as overdependent, passive, inhibited and showing compulsive tendencies.

However, the mentioned concepts were developed on the basis of observations made in highly selected patient groups. This explains why subsequent attempts to test their validity, or to simply find out whether the underlying observations could be made also in other patients with the disease, failed. Feldman et al.[5] compared 34 unselected hospitalized patients with ulcerative colitis with 74 consecutive patients hospitalized for gastrointestinal illnesses not affecting the large bowel. Each patient had two standard psychiatric interviews of the free-association type and the amount of psychiatric time spent with and discussing each patient was, on the average, 10–12 hours. The evaluation included descriptive and dynamic variables, such as symptoms, cognition, ego strength, defensiveness, acting out, dependence, external problems, attitude towards illness, anxiety, depression, personality type, background and family interrelationships. It was found that as many as possible of the emotional factors relating to psychosomatic illness mentioned in the literature did *not* apply in any significant degree and that patients with ulcerative colitis showed abnormalities no more frequently than did patients of the control group. In the same way, Feldman and co-workers[6] studied 19 consecutive unselected patients with Crohn's disease. Again, no evidence was found that an emotional factor was of a significant aetiological importance. In a study by Helzer et al.[7], 50 consecutive patients with ulcerative colitis were found not to differ in their personality profiles and their obsessionality from patients with other chronic, but non-gastrointestinal, medical illnesses.

STRESSFUL LIFE EVENTS

Another widespread notion is that onset and exacerbation of ulcerative colitis were closely related to stressful events in the patient's life. One of the advocates of this notion was Engel[8], who stated in 1973: 'When one carefully studies the setting in which symptoms develop and remit, there is a clear-cut relationship between psychological stress and onset and exacerbation on the one hand and psychological support and remission on the other'. Subsequent research, however, was unable to confirm such a relationship. Feldman et al.[5] could not find any examples of significant separation experiences or anxieties in 34 unselected hospitalized patients with ulcerative colitis. The onset of the disease was preceded by a moderate-to-severe degree of stress in only five and the relapse in only nine of their cases, and no other relative frequency of such precipitating factors was observed in the 74 patients of the control group. In a subsequent study, the same authors[6] found that the occurrence of precipitating factors in 19 patients suffering from Crohn's disease was less than in unselected patients who had been hospitalized for other medical reasons.

No support for the notion that a characteristic constellation of events underlay the onset of symptoms in a susceptible population could be found in the epidemiologic studies of Mendeloff, Monk and co-workers[9,10]. These investigations found that events, which might be considered as disruptive, emotionally or psychologically, were reported to very similar extents by 158 patients with ulcerative colitis and 69 with Crohn's disease, by 105 patients with irritable colon syndrome and by 753 individuals out of the general population. Sessions *et al.*[11] reported that, in 47 patients with Crohn's disease, life stress, as reported in the Holmes–Rahe Schedule of Recent Experience, was not clearly correlated with disease activity. No correlations between the frequency of potentially stressful life events occurring within the six months prior to an interview and the severity of ulcerative colitis and Crohn's disease at that time were found in other studies[7,12] either. Rampton and co-workers[13] observed that emotional stress was no more frequent in eleven patients with ulcerative colitis in the four weeks preceding a relapse than in 50 patients with no relapse. Interestingly, in the patients with relapses, there was a high prevalence of intake of prostaglandin synthetase inhibitors, including paracetamol.

Also, in a *prospective* study extending over one year in 22 patients with ulcerative colitis, no correlation between the incidence of stressful life events and either symptomatic deterioration or objectively defined relapse of the disease could be detected[14]. Furthermore, patients with anxiety and psychoneurosis ratings in the upper range of normal did not relapse more frequently. Consonant results were obtained in a recently published prospective study extending over two years[15]: in 48 patients with ulcerative colitis and in 16 with Crohn's disease, changes in symptoms correlated poorly with self-reported life events, and the correlation did not become better when symptom changes were lagged behind the occurrence of life events by up to two months. Furthermore, the frequency of stressful events was not increased in the periods preceding an exacerbation.

Thus, the available data do not speak in favour of the notion that stressful life events influence the natural history of inflammatory bowel disease. However, an exacerbation of the illness may itself precipitate a depressive reaction or a disruption in the patient's adjustment to his environment and interfere with his ability to fight the disease.

PSYCHIATRIC DISEASE

A series of studies has shown that patients with inflammatory bowel disease are no more likely to receive a psychiatric diagnosis or to exhibit neurotic traits than are patients with other chronic diseases and even healthy individuals. Sloan *et al.*[16], who reviewed 2000 cases with ulcerative colitis treated at the Mayo Clinic between 1918 and 1937, found no increased incidence of psychoneurosis. Goldberg[17] observed that patients suffering from Crohn's disease had no higher frequency of psychiatric symptoms than patients with idiopathic steatorrhoea and lactose intolerance. Others observed that patients with ulcerative colitis were no more anxious than healthy individuals[14,18], and that the severity of Crohn's disease was not correlated with either anxiety or depression[11]. In a study in children and adolescents, significant behaviour disorders or neurosis were found in only eight out of 87 with ulcerative colitis and six out of 61 with Crohn's disease, and psychosocial problems in the immediate household in only nine with colitis and thirteen with Crohn's disease, i.e. in about the frequencies to be expected in any chronic disease[19]. In 50 consecutive patients with ulcerative colitis, no greater incidence of psychiatric disorder was observed than in patients with chronic non-gastrointestinal illnesses[7] and the seriousness of the psychiatric disorder was not related to the severity of colitis. Patients with Crohn's disease, however, met diagnostic criteria for some psychiatric disorder at some time in their life more often than patients with other chronic illnesses, although the severities of Crohn's disease and psychiatric disorders appeared to be independent of one another[12].

Alpers and co-workers[20] found that depression was no more common in 50 consecutive patients with ulcerative colitis and 50 with Crohn's disease than in 50 patients with other chronic medical diseases, and that the severity of the inflammatory bowel disease was not affected by the onset of psychiatric disease. In a recent study, the prevalence of psychiatric disorder was observed not to be increased before and after the onset of ulcerative colitis, but to be higher in patients with Crohn's disease[21]. No such differing prevalence of psychiatric disorder in the two disorders was found in a study in 71 patients with ulcerative colitis and 91 with Crohn's disease, which also revealed no significant association between the presence of psychiatric and physical illness; ongoing psychiatric illness, however, adversely affected physical recovery[22].

PSYCHOTHERAPY?

The supposed importance of psychological factors for the development and the course of inflammatory bowel disease fostered the hope that psychotherapeutic interventions aimed at removing these harmful factors could cure, or at least help to cure, the disease. Grace *et al.*[23] reported a study in which 34 patients with ulcerative colitis were treated for at least two years with psychoanalytically oriented individual and/or group therapy in addition to their medical care. Thirty-four other patients, who were matched for age and sex as well as for severity and duration of illness, received only medical care. It was found that, of the patients with additional psychotherapy, 22 could be considered as cured or improved, whereas this was the case in only 11 patients having received only medical treatment. However, the authors did not state how the patients were allotted to the two treatment groups and the outcome of therapy was not assessed blindly. The therapeutic study by O'Connor, Karush and co-workers[24,25], which has received great attention, can be regarded, by current standards, as having anecdotal value only. Fifty-seven individuals with ulcerative colitis, who had been referred for psychosis, personality disorder or psychoneurosis, were treated, in addition to their medical care, with analytically oriented psychotherapy over a 7-year period. Retrospectively, these patients, all but one of whom had a psychiatric diagnosis, were matched with 57 other patients, of whom only 20 had a psychiatric diagnosis. It was found that the incidence of medical failure, namely colectomy, and of mortality was about the same in the two groups, whereas the clinical gradings of diseases were slightly better in the patients with additional psychotherapy. The authors concluded that psychotherapy had a favourable effect on the course of the disease, although there was no direct relationship between the degrees of physical and psychological improvement.

The only psychotherapeutic study meeting current standards is one in which eighty non-hospitalized patients were randomly assigned to two treatment groups[26]. One group received medical treatment only, whereas the other also received a stress management programme consisting of teaching a relaxation technique, personal planning skills and communication techniques. Patients were followed up at 4-monthly intervals for one year by interviewers who were blind to the patients' group designation. It was found that, in the group with additional stress management training, the Crohn's Disease Activity Index decreased, together with an improvement in physical and psychosocial well-being, whereas, in the group with medical treatment only, no such effects were noted. Although it is not possible to extrapolate from these results to the effects the stress management training might have on the illness course over longer periods of time, they indicate that such interventions may be suited to increase the patients' ability to cope with the disease and, thereby, to decrease their functional disability. Functional disabilities may represent a serious problem, despite the fact that many studies have shown that patients with inflammatory bowel disease actually do not differ from healthy individuals in their social and physical activities[27,31]. With regard to children, Hamilton et al.[19] observed in their case 'a superb capacity to adapt' and that the afflicted children, as well as their parents, continued to perform adequately despite severe illness. They further observed that, 'emotionally, the families seemed to function best when the parents maintained a supportive relationship with the child, while also keeping enough distance to avoid pushing the child into the role of an invalid'.

Psychotherapeutic interventions, of course, may also be useful to help the patients to deal with their rightful concerns about having an ostomy bag, having surgery, losing bowel control, developing cancer, etc.[32] They may also be directed at encouraging patients not to perceive themselves as sick but as 'different' and to take a more active role in the management of their disease. In patients maintaining the 'sick role' for fear of losing benefits, such as increased attention from their environment or work relief, treatment can be directed at helping them to return to 'well' behaviour. Also, however, much more pedestrian approaches, such as to encourage the patient to participate in a self-help organization, may yield great benefit. Self-help organizations can provide a social reference group, in which information and coping strategies can be shared, and increased reliance on the self is fostered. Most important for the patients is to have some understanding of their disease, of why they feel unwell, have pain or diarrhoea, and of why they should undergo investigations and comply with their scheduled treatment.

In conclusion, the original psychosomatic concepts that a specific unconscious conflict, a specific type of interpersonal relationship or other psychological factors could predispose an individual to the development of physical illness, which implied that such illness must also be psychologically preventable, could not be substantiated by empirical studies. However, psychosocial factors may be important determinants for the patients' reaction to and their handling of the disease, and thus should not escape the physician's attention.

References

1. Alexander, F. (1950). *Psychosomatic Medicine: Its Principles and Applications*. (New York: Norton)
2. Grace, W.J. and Graham, D.T. (1952). Relationship of specific attitudes and emotions to certain bodily diseases. *Psychsom. Med.*, **14**, 243–251
3. Engel, G.L. (1955). Studies of ulcerative colitis. III. The nature of the psychologic processes. *Am. J. Med.*, **19**, 231–256
4. McDermott, J. and Finch, S. (1967). Ulcerative colitis in children. *J. Am. Acad. Child Psychiatr.*, **6**, 512–517
5. Feldman, F., Cantor, D., Soll, S. and Bachrach, W. (1967). Psychiatric study of a consecutive series of 34 patients with ulcerative colitis. *Br. Med. J.*, **3**, 14–17
6. Feldman, F., Cantor, D., Soll, S. and Bachrach, W. (1967). Psychiatric study of a consecutive series of 19 patients with regional ileitis. *Br. Med. J.*, **4**, 711–714
7. Helzer, J.E., Stillings, W.A., Chammas, S., Norland, C.C. and Alpers, D.H. (1982). A controlled study of the association between ulcerative colitis and psychiatric diagnoses. *Dig. Dis. Sci.*, **27**, 513–518
8. Engel, G.L. (1973). Ulcerative colitis. In Lindner, A.E. (ed.) *Emotional Factors in Gastrointestinal Illness*, pp. 99–112. (Amsterdam: Excerpta Medica)
9. Mendeloff, A.I., Monk, M., Siegel, C.I. and Lilienfeld, A. (1970). Illness experience and life stresses in patients with irritable colon and with ulcerative colitis. An epidemiologic study of ulcerative colitis and regional enteritis in Baltimore, 1960–1964. *N. Engl. J. Med.*, **282**, 14–17
10. Monk, M., Mendeloff, A.I., Siegel, C.I. and Lilienfeld, A. (1970). An epidemiological study of ulcerative colitis and regional enteritis among adults in Baltimore – III. Psychological and possible stress-precipitating factors. *J. Chron. Dis.*, **22**, 565–578
11. Sessions, J.T., Raft, D. and Tate, S. (1978). The severity of Crohn's disease does not correlate with life stress, depression and anxiety (abstract). *Gastroenterology*, **74**, 1144
12. Helzer, J.E., Chammas, S., Norland, C.C., Stillings, W.A. and Alpers, D.H. (1984). A study of the association between Crohn's disease and psychiatric illness. *Gastroenterology*, **86**, 324–330
13. Rampton, D.S., McNeil, N.I. and Sarner, M. (1982). Events preceding relapse in ulcerative colitis (abstract). *Gut*, **23**, 434–435
14. Campbell, D., Shannon, S. and Collins, S.M. (1986). The relationship between personality, stress and disease activity in ulcerative colitis (abstract). *Gastroenterology*, **90**, 1364
15. North, C.S., Clouse, R.E., Helzer, J.E., Spitznagel, E. and Alpers, D.H. (1989). Inflammatory bowel disease (IBD), life events, and depression: a prospective study (abstract). *Gastroenterology*, **96**, A367
16. Sloan, W.P., Bargen, J.A. and Gage, R.P. (1950). Life histories of patients with chronic ulcerative colitis: a review of 2,000 cases. *Gastroenterology*, **16**, 25–37
17. Goldberg, D. (1970). A psychiatric study of patients with diseases of the small intestine, *Gut*, **11**, 459–465

18. Esler, M.D. and Goulston, K.J. (1973). Levels of anxiety in colonic disorders. *N. Engl. J. Med.*, **288**, 16–20
19. Hamilton, J.R., Bruce, G.A., Abdourhaman, M. and Gall, D.G. (1979). Inflammatory bowel disease in children and adolescents. *Adv. Pediatr.*, **26**, 311–341
20. Alpers, D.H., Norland, C.C., Stillings, W.A., Chamnes, S. and Helzer, J.E. (1980). Increased prevalence of psychiatric disease in Crohn's disease (CD) but not ulcerative colitis (UC) (abstract). *Gastroenterology*, **78**, 1131
21. Tarter, R.E., Switala, J., Carra, J., Edwards, K.L. and Van Thiel, D.H. (1987). Inflammatory bowel disease: psychiatric status of patients before and after disease onset. *Int. J. Psychiatr. Med.*, **17**, 173–181
22. Andrews, H., Barczak, P. and Allan, R.N. (1987). Psychiatric illness in patients with inflammatory bowel disease. *Gut*, **28**, 1600–1604
23. Grace, W.J., Pinsky, R.H. and Wolff, H.G. (1954). The treatment of ulcerative colitis. II. *Gastroenterology*, **26**, 462–468
24. O'Connor, J.F., Daniels, G., Flood, C., Karush, A., Moses, L. and Stern, L.O. (1964). An evaluation of the effectiveness of psychotherapy in the treatment of ulcerative colitis. *Ann. Intern. Med.*, **60**, 587–602
25. Karush, A., Daniels, G.E., O'Connor, J.F. and Stern, L.O. (1968). The response to psychotherapy in chronic ulcerative colitis. I. Pretreatment factors. *Psychosom. Med.*, **30**, 255–276
26. Milne, B., Joachim, G. and Niedhardt, J. (1986). A stress management programme for inflammatory bowel disease patients. *J. Adv. Nurs.*, **11**, 561–567
27. Hendriksen, C. and Binder, V. (1980). Social prognosis in patients with ulcerative colitis. *Br. Med. J.*, **281**, 581–583
28. Joachim, G. and Milne, B. (1987). Inflammatory bowel disease: effects on lifestyle. *J. Adv. Nurs.*, **12**, 483–487
29. Sørensen, V.Z., Olsen, B.G. and Binder, V. (1987). Life prospects and quality of life in patients with Crohn's disease. *Gut*, **28**, 382–385
30. Bellanger, J., Le Quintrec, Y. and Alle, J.P. (1987). Le vécu de la maladie de Crohn. Etude par quéstionnaire. *Ann. Gastroentérol. Hepatol. (Paris)*, **23**, 221–227
31. Feurle, G.E., Keller, O., Hassels, K. and Jesdinsky, H.J. (1983). Soziale Auswirkungen des Morbus Crohn. *Dtsch. Med. Wochenschr.*, **108**, 971–975
32. Drossman, D.A., Patrick, D.L., Mitchell, C.M. and Zagami, E.A. (1988). What are the disease related concerns of patients with IBD? (abstract). *Gastroenterology*, **94**, A104

Section II
Coeliac disease

13
Management of coeliac disease in children: a personal view

J.A. WALKER-SMITH

Aretaeus the Cappodocian, the distinguished Greek physician of antiquity, wrote in the first century concerning the treatment of the coeliac affection that he recommended "drinks taken before meals, for otherwise bread is very little conducive to trim vigour"[30]. However, despite the enthusiasts, Aretaeus, although wise, was scarcely so prescient as to anticipate the role of gluten.

Likewise, Gee, writing in 1888, stated that "to regulate food is the main part of treatment", and concluded his classic report with the words, "But if the patient can be cured at all, it must be by means of a diet."[31]

However, it was Dicke, in 1950, who recognized the role of wheat flour and then gluten in particular in this disease[32]. Then it was Margot Shiner in 1957 who placed the diagnosis on a firm basis by describing the characteristic mucosal lesion on biopsy[33].

INITIAL MANAGEMENT

The initial management of coeliac disease in childhood is: in the first instance, making a provisional diagnosis of coeliac disease based upon solid evidence; second, instituting therapy with a gluten-free diet; third, demonstrating a clinical response to this diet. Subsequent management, in particular the need for a gluten challenge in every case, and the need for a gluten-free diet for life, continues to be a matter of some debate. However, it is clear that, in the management of coeliac disease, diagnosis and treatment proceed side by side.

The initial provisional diagnosis of coeliac disease in a child with appropriate clinical features should be based upon the demonstration of an abnormal small intestinal mucosa with features characteristic of untreated coeliac disease using the technique of small intestinal biopsy. This features a flat mucosa on dissecting microscopy and hyperplastic villous atrophy on

147

Table 1 Diagnostic criteria for coeliac disease (ESPGAN criteria)

Abnormal small intestinal mucosa (usually flat)
Clinical response to a gluten-free diet
Histological response to a gluten-free diet
Histological clinical relapse following gluten challenge

light microscopy. This is followed by showing a clinical response to the withdrawal of gluten from the child's diet. A clinical response is demonstrated when there is significant weight gain and relief of all symptoms of the disease.

GLUTEN CHALLENGE

Some paediatricians would then consider the diagnosis of coeliac disease to have been established. However, reintroduction of gluten into the child's diet at a later date, i.e. gluten challenge or provocation when the small intestinal mucosa has been shown to return to normal, followed by mucosal deterioration with or without a clinical relapse, is regarded as necessary by other paediatricians before the diagnosis of coeliac disease may be said to have been definitively, i.e. finally and unequivocally, established. Such a relapse in mucosal appearance may not occur for up to 2 years, or sometimes much longer, after the reintroduction of gluten into the child's diet.

These diagnostic criteria for coeliac disease are listed in Table 1. These criteria are sometimes known as the Interlaken or ESPGAN Criteria because they arose from a meeting of the European Society for Paediatric Gastroenterology in Interlaken in 1969[1]. With some modifications, these criteria have stood the test of time and continue to be a valuable guide to diagnosis[2]. Yet they have now been challenged by Guandalini et al.[3] who used these criteria in the remarkable number of 2400 children to establish the diagnosis of coeliac disease.

The author's view, enunciated first in 1975, again in 1979 and 1988[4-6], is in accord with the view of Guandalini et al.[3] that these criteria, in practice, do not need to be fulfilled in every case diagnosed as coeliac disease. In fact, most children diagnosed as having coeliac disease do not need a gluten challenge. In a series of 192 children diagnosed as having coeliac disease at Queen Elizabeth Hospital between 1960 and 1985[7], only 81 fulfilled the ESPGAN criteria (41%).

Indications for gluten challenge

A child previously diagnosed as suffering from ceoliac disease and having a gluten-free diet requires reinvestigation in order to fulfil these criteria in only three particular situations.

(1) If there is any doubt about the original diagnosis. This is particularly

Table 2 Reported causes of a flat mucosa

Coeliac disease, i.e. permanent gluten intolerance
Transient gluten intolerance ⎫ Temporary
Cows' milk-sensitive enteropathy ⎬ food sensitive
Soy protein intolerance ⎭ enteropathies
Gastroenteritis and postenteritis syndrome
Giardiasis
Autoimmune enteropathy
Acquired hypogammaglobulinaemia
Tropical sprue
Protein energy malnutrition

---

necessary if the child was started on such a diet without a previous small intestinal biopsy or if the initial biopsy was diagnostically inadequate or the mucosal abnormality was in some way uncharacteristic.

(2) If the child was less than 2 years of age at the time of diagnosis. Although a flat small intestinal mucosa is characteristic of coeliac disease, there are a number of other causes of such a mucosal abnormality in infancy and early childhood (Table 2). Indeed, the mean age of the 155 children, in Guandalini *et al.*'s study, where the diagnosis of coeliac disease was not confirmed, was 8 months. The differential diagnosis of coeliac disease is thus a problem of infancy.

(3) If the child or teenager himself wishes to abandon the diet, a controlled gluten challenge is preferable to an uncontrolled challenge.

ANALYSIS OF THE INITIAL DIAGNOSTIC BIOPSY

Although these other causes of a flat mucosa do exist there are important morphometric differences between them. For example, the flat mucosa found occasionally in severe cases of cow's milk-sensitive enteropathy and also in the postenteritis enteropathies are typically thin mucosae whereas the flat mucosa found in coeliac disease is the same thickness as normal, although it is flat[8].

Analysis of intraepithelial lymphocytes gives invaluable diagnostic information. Recent studies of the intraepithelial lymphoid population of patients with coeliac disease now open up the prospect of one single diagnostic biopsy being adequate to make the final diagnosis of coeliac disease. It now seems probable that there is a unique change in this population which is specific to coeliac disease patients, both treated and untreated.

ANALYSIS OF INTRAEPITHELIAL LYMPHOCYTES

For some time, the intraepithelial lymphocyte count, i.e. the density of lymphocytes in relation to epithelial cells, has been regarded as being diagnostically useful both in adults with coeliac disease and in children with coeliac disease[9]. It has been especially useful for assessing the response of the mucosa on biopsy to gluten elimination and challenge. Some doubt concerning the value of this measurement has been cast by the work of Marsh[10]. He has related the number of lymphocytes in the epithelium of the small intestine to a constant square of muscularis mucosae. Using this technique, the absolute number of lymphocytes actually falls because of the dramatic reduction in surface area in untreated coeliac disease. Theoretically and conceptually, this is of great interest but does nothing to detract from the diagnostic value of the intraepithelial lymphocyte count as a practical tool where a rise in density is a feature of active coeliac disease.

However, other disease states are associated with an increased intra-epithelial lymphocyte count, e.g. in adults, untreated dermatitis herpetiformis, tropical sprue and giardiasis and also in some children with giardiasis, cow's milk-sensitive enteropathy and unexplained diarrhoea with failure to thrive[11]. Thus this change in intraepithelial lymphocyte density is not specific.

In recent times, the distinctive nature of the intraepithelial lymphocytes as a compartment of gut-associated lymphoid tissue has become apparent. It has in fact been the use of monoclonal antibodies to study the surface markers of these cells that has opened up the following question. Is there a specific change in intraepithelial lymphocytes in coeliac disease? It has, for example, been shown that by far the great majority of intraepithelial lymphocytes in normal human small bowel mucosa react with an antibody to human lymphocytes and that most of these are of the suppressor-cytotoxic phenotype[12]. Thus, in modern terminology, it has been established that the intraepithelial lymphocyte is predominantly a T cell which expresses the CD3 trimer which is an antigen associated with all forms of the T cell receptor and also CD8, which is an antigen associated with MHC class I restricted T cell.

Double immunoenzymatic staining has been used now to define new intraepithelial lymphocyte subpopulations in man and to look specifically at coeliac disease, both treated and untreated. Using this technique, Spencer et al.[13] found that, in normal small intestinal mucosa, 6% of the intraepithelial T cells which expressed CD3 did not express T cell subset antigens CD4 or CD8. This population of cells is often called the subset negative cells[14]. In coeliac disease, the percentage of these CD3+,CD4-,CD8- cells increases to 28%, a highly significant increase from the normal finding of 6%. Furthermore, this change was found not only in adults and children with untreated coeliac disease but in adults on a gluten-free diet with a normal mucosa. However, it also occurred in the mucosae of adult patients with enteropathy-associated T cell lymphoma but did not occur in other patients with small intestinal enteropathy. So, in coeliac disease, there is a highly specific increase in density of CD3 positive, CD4 negative and CD8 negative intraepithelial lymphocytes.

Looking further at this change in intraepithelial lymphocytes (IEL) in coeliac disease, the T cell receptor expressed by these cells has been investigated. CD3+,CD4-,CD8- T cells, i.e. the subset negative cells,

Table 3 Expression of TCR δ by intraepithelial lymphocytes

Normal small intestinal mucosa	11%
Coeliac disease	33%
Tropical sprue	5%
Cow's milk-sensitive enteropathy	14.6%
Postenteritis syndrome	34.7%
Autoimmune enteropathy	6.3%

express the γ/δ hetero dimer rather than the usual α/β hetero dimer as their antigen receptor. So the spotlight has turned to those intraepithelial lymphocytes which express T cell receptor γ/δ in coeliac disease.

Spencer et al.[15] have used immunocytochemistry to study this issue using monoclonal antibody to δ chain of the T cell receptor TCR δ1. Children and adults with enteropathies of diverse cause, namely tropical sprue, cow's milk-sensitive enteropathy, postenteritis syndrome and autoimmune entero-pathy, have been compared with coeliac disease (Table 3). 33% of IEL in coeliac disease express TCR δ1 compared with 11% in normal mucosa and comparable percentages in abnormal mucosae except one case of postenter-itis syndrome. In this one case, however, unlike coeliac disease, the overall intraepithelial lymphocyte count was not increased.

Further work is clearly required in a wide range of disease controls but, at present, from the data of Spencer et al., it seems clear that there is a highly characteristic abnormality of the intraepithelial lymphocyte population in both untreated and treated patients with coeliac disease, both adults and children. This observation has been confirmed by Savilahti et al.[16].

The way is now open for monoclonal antibody analysis of the intra-epithelial lymphocyte population of abnormal small intestinal mucosae to be a specific diagnostic test, made on a single small intestinal biopsy. If this becomes true, sequential biopsies, as currently required to fulfil the ESPGAN criteria, will no longer be required. However, the initial diagnostic small intestinal biopsy will remain as important as ever.

TRANSIENT GLUTEN INTOLERANCE

In the age group under two years, there exists a syndrome known as transient gluten intolerance[17,18] as opposed to permanent gluten intolerance, i.e. coeliac disease. There has not yet been an opportunity to analyse the intraepithelial lymphocytes in these children for γ/δ expression.

In Western countries, the great majority of children with a flat small intestinal mucosa, and especially those who respond to a gluten-free diet, do have coeliac disease. However, in infants under the age of 2 years, there is a significant possibility that the child with a flat small intestinal mucosa and a clinical response to a gluten-free diet has a cause other than coeliac disease. In a series of 218 children initially diagnosed as coeliac disease, 26 did not relapse after challenge (11.9%) despite an initial abnormal mucosa and response to a gluten-free diet[7]; all were under two years of age at presentation. Hence, the advice given is to reinvestigate children under two years at some point later in childhood with serial biopsies related to elimination and challenge.

CIRCULATING ANTIBODIES

Gliadin antibodies, in particular IgA antibodies, as well as the presence of antireticulin and antiendomysial antibodies may provide information of diagnostic usefulness and are a way to analyse response to elimination and challenge with gluten[19]. However, disease controls can be positive[20]. This test cannot be relied on by itself as elevated titres of gliadin antibodies may occur in other enteropathies[21]. At Queen Elizabeth Hospital, however, on the only occasions where gliadin antibodies have not been detected in untreated coeliac disease, reticulin antibodies have been positive[21]. Nevertheless, the advice must remain that the initial small bowel biopsy is essential for diagnosis.

Enthusiasm for this serological approach has come from communities where there are not significant numbers of non-coeliac disease controls and, as a result, circulating antibodies have largely been used in these studies to separate coeliac from normal individuals. This is not to deny that these tests, when abnormal, are strong pointers to the diagnosis of coeliac disease in communities where small intestinal biopsy is not available; their presence at least shows that coeliac disease is possible. However, in communities, for example the Sudan[22] and India[23], where small intestinal mucosal damage, especially as a sequel to gastroenteritis, is so common, it is only by use of the ESPGAN criteria that incontrovertible evidence has been provided that coeliac disease does exist and is the cause of small intestinal mucosal damage in individual children, although antibodies may provide useful information when biopsy is unavailable.

TECHNIQUE OF GLUTEN CHALLENGE OR PROVOCATION

Gluten challenge may be carried out in the following manner. A small intestinal biopsy is performed while the child is still on a gluten-free diet in order to demonstrate that the mucosa is in fact normal or near normal. If such a preliminary biopsy is abnormal, this suggests that the child has coeliac disease and is not keeping strictly to a gluten-free diet, or that some other disease is present so further investigations may be necessary. Usually, such a biopsy is normal when the child has been on a gluten-free diet for 2 years or more. Reinvestigation of a child with the typical features of coeliac disease after a period of less than 2 years on a gluten-free diet is not usually indicated.

Once a normal mucosa has been demonstrated, the child is given a normal diet containing gluten, or gluten powder is added to his gluten-free diet. Gluten powder may be given to avoid the upset to a child produced by changing his gluten-free diet which has already been in use for some time. If the child does return to a 'normal' diet, care must be taken to ensure that he does in fact eat gluten-containing foods. A regular check by a dietitian of his daily wheat intake in grams per day is very useful. The author prefers such a return to a normal diet rather than the use of gluten powder. Should significant symptoms ensue after a gluten challenge, a further biopsy is performed after an interval of a week following the return of such symptoms. If the mucosa is then abnormal, the diagnosis of coeliac disease may be said to have been established, i.e. a histological relapse has occurred on reintroduction of gluten to the diet. It is not necessary for the mucosa to be flat to diagnose such a relapse; the presence of significant mucosal abnormalities, for example increased plasma cells and lymphocytes in the lamina propria and abnormalities of the surface enterocytes, and especially a rise in the intraepithelial lymphocyte count, is sufficient. This latter measurement is particularly useful diagnostically.

Even if symptoms fail to occur, small intestinal biopsy should be performed in any event after 3 months' exposure to gluten since histological relapse may precede clinical relapse. If the mucosa is then still normal, the child is observed and kept on a normal diet or a diet with added gluten and another biopsy is performed should symptoms subsequently develop. If symptoms do not develop, a further biopsy is done after 2 years' exposure to gluten. If the mucosa is abnormal, the diagnosis is coeliac disease, but, if normal, then coeliac disease is most unlikely. However, the precise period of 2 years is somewhat arbitrary. There are now a few children reported in the literature who have taken longer than 2 years to relapse, sometimes several years[24,25].

Serial estimation of gliadin antibodies related to gluten elimination and challenge following the demonstration of a flat mucosa and a response to a gluten-free diet is a diagnostic strategy which could avoid serial biopsies or else indicate their appropriate timings, but it does not avoid the need for the initial small intestinal biopsy which demonstrates characteristic pathology, i.e. a flat mucosa on dissecting microscopy and hyperplastic villous atrophy histologically. Failure to do this may lead to the performance some years later of these extensive investigations, only to show that the child did not have coeliac disease in the first place and so did not need a gluten-free diet at all.

DURATION OF A GLUTEN-FREE DIET IN COELIAC DISEASE

In the author's view, this should be life-long, i.e. permanent. In the short term, this will permit normal growth with achievement of full growth potential[27]. In the long term, a gluten-free diet may prevent malignancy complicating coeliac disease. Early studies, e.g. that of Holmes et al.[28], failed to show any protection against the risk of malignancy in adults by the use of a gluten-free diet. However, recently, a long-term study from the same group[29] has reported a definite benefit from a gluten-free diet. For patients with coeliac disease who have taken a gluten-free diet for five years or more, the risk of developing cancer was not increased when compared with the general population. Those taking a reduced gluten or a normal diet had increased risk of cancers of the mouth, pharynx and oesophagus and also of lymphoma. These results provide compelling evidence for advising patients to adhere to a strict gluten-free diet for life.

The hypothesis that the enteropathy in enteropathy-associated T cell lymphoma is due to coeliac disease is supported by the observation that the various intraepithelial lymphocyte populations in both enteropathies are indistinguishable[13] as mentioned earlier. This adds further weight to the argument for a strict gluten-free diet for life, as one could speculate that the tendency of patients with enteropathy-associated T cell lymphoma to develop malignancy may be related to chronic activation of cells in the mucosa by continuous gluten intake.

CONCLUSION

The management of coeliac disease centres upon accurate diagnosis and the need for a life-long gluten-free diet.

References

1. Meeuwisse, G.W. (1970). Diagnostic criteria in coeliac disease. *Acta Paediatr. Scand.*, **59**, 461
2. McNeish, A.S., Harms, K., Ray, J., Shmerling, D. H. and Walker-Smith, J. A. (1979). Re-evaluation of diagnostic criteria for coeliac disease. *Arch. Dis. Child.*, **54**, 783
3. Guandalini, S., Ventura, A., Ansaldi, N., Guinta, A.M., Greco, L., Lazzari, R., Mastella, G. and Rubino, A. (1989). Diagnosis of coeliac disease: time for a change? *Arch. Dis. Child.*, **64**, 1320-1325
4. Walker-Smith, J.A. (1975). *Diseases of the Small Intestine in Childhood*, 1st Edn. (London: Pitman Medical)
5. Walker-Smith, J.A. (1979). *Diseases of the Small Intestine in Childhood*, 2nd Edn. (London: Pitman Medical)
6. Walker-Smith, J.A. (1988). *Diseases of the Small Intestine in Childhood*, 3rd Edn. (London: Butterworths)
7. Kelly, D., Phillips, A.D., Elliott, E.J., Dias, J.A. and Walker-Smith, J.A. (1988). The rise and fall of coeliac disease 1960-1985. *Arch. Dis. Child.*, **64**, 1157-1160
8. Maluenda, C., Phillips, A.D., Briddon, A. and Walker-Smith, J.A. (1984). Quantitive analysis of small intestinal mucosa in cow's milk sensitive enteropathy. *J. Paediatr. Gastroenterol. Nutr.*, **3**, 349-357
9. Ferguson, A. and Murray, D. (1971). Quantitation of intraepithelial lymphocytes in human jejunum. *Gut*, **129**, 88
10. Marsh, M.N. (1985). Functional and structural aspects of the epithelial lymphocyte with implications for coeliac disease and tropical sprue. *Scand. J. Gastroenterol.*, **114**, 55-75
11. Phillips, A.D., Rice, S.J., France, N.E. and Walker-Smith, J.A. (1979). Small intestinal lymphocyte levels in cow's milk protein intolerance. *Gut*, **20**, 509
12. Selby, W.S., Janossy, G. and Jewell, D.P. (1981). Immunohistological characterization of intraepithelial lymphocytes of the human gastrointestinal tract. *Gut*, **22**, 169
13. Spencer, J., MacDonald, T.T., Diss, T.C., Walker-Smith, J.A., Ciclitira, P.J. and Isaacson, P.G. (1989). Changes in intraepithelial lymphocyte subpopulations in coeliac disease and enteropathy associated T cell lymphoma (malignant histiocytosis of the intestine). *Gut*, **30**, 339
14. Jenkins, D., Goodall, A. and Scott, B.B. (1989). T lymphocyte populations in normal and coeliac mucosa defined by monoclonal antibodies. *Gut*, **30**, 339

15. Spencer, J., MacDonald, T.T., Isaacson, P.G. and Walker-Smith, J.A. (1989). T cell receptor expression by human intraepithelial lymphocytes: differences between coeliac disease and normal jejunal biopsies and non-coeliac enteropathy. *Pediatr. Res.,* **3,** 279
16. Savilhati, E. (1990). Increased gamma/delta cells in celiacs. *Pediatr. Res.* (in press)
17. Walker-Smith, J.A. (1970). Transient gluten intolerance. *Arch. Dis. Child.* **45,** 523–526
18. Walker-Smith, J.A. (1987). Transient gluten intolerance: does it exist? *Neth. J. Med.,* **31,** 269–278
19. Burgin-Wolff, A., Gaze, H., Lentze, M. and Nussle, D. (1990). Gliadin and endomysium antibody determinations in childhood coeliac disease. In Kumar, P. and Walker-Smith, J.A. (eds.) *Proceedings of International Coeliac Symposium* (London)
20. Unsworth, D.J. and Walker-Smith, J.A. (1983). Antigliadin and anti-reticulin antibodies in childhood coeliac disease. *Lancet,* **2,** 874–875
21. Dias, J., Unsworth, D.J. and Walker-Smith, J.A. (1987). Antigliadin and anti-reticulin antibodies in screening for coeliac disease. *Lancet,* **2,** 157–158
22. Suliman, G.I. (1978). Coeliac disease in Sudanese children. *Gut,* **19,** 121
23. Khoshoo, V., Bhan, M.K., Unsworth, D.J., Kumar, R. and Walker-Smith, J.A. (1988). Anti-reticulin antibodies: useful adjunct to histopathology in diagnosing coeliac disease, especially in a developing country. *J. Pediatr. Gastroenterol. Nutr.,* **7,** 864–866
24. Egan-Mitchell, B., Fottress, P.F. and McNicholl, B. (1978). Prolonged gluten intolerance in treated coeliac disease. In McNicholl, B., McCarthy, C.F. and Fottrell, P.F. (eds.) *Perspectives in Coeliac Disease,* pp. 251–259 (Lancaster: MTP Press)
25. Polanco, I. and Larrauri, J. (1990). Does transient gluten intolerance exist indeed? In Kumar, P. and Walker-Smith, J.A. (eds.) *Proceedings of International Coeliac Symposium.* (London)
26. Schmitz, J., Jos, J. and Rey, J. (1978). Transient mucosal atrophy in confirmed coeliac disease. In McNicholl, B., McCarthy, C.F. and Fottrell, P.F. (eds.) *Perspectives in Coeliac Disease,* p. 259 (Lancaster: MTP Press)
27. Kumar, P.J., Walker-Smith, J.A., Milla, P., Harria, G., Colyer, J. and Halliday, R. (1988). The teenage coeliac: follow-up study of 102 patients. *Arch. Dis. Child.,* **63** 916–920
28. Holmes, G.K.T., Stokes, P.L., Sorahan, T.M., Prior, P., Waterhouse, J.A.H.M. and Cooke, W.T. (1976). Coeliac disease, gluten-free diet and malignancy. *Gut,* **17,** 612
29. Holmes, G.K.T., Prior, P., Lane, M.R., Pope, D. and Allan, R.N. (1989). Malignancy in coeliac disease - effect of a gluten-free diet. *Gut,* **30,** 336–339
30. Adams, F. (1856). *The Extant Works of Aretaeus the Cappadocian.* (London: The Sydenham Society)
31. Gee, S.J. (1888). On the coeliac affection. *St. Bartholomew's Hospital Reports,* **24,** 17
32. Dicke, W.K. (1950). *Coeliakie: een onderzoek naar de nadelige invloed van sommige graansoorte op de lijder aan coeliakie.* MD Thesis, Utrecht
33. Sakula, J. and Siner, M. (1957). Coeliac disease with atrophy of the small intestine mucosa. *Lancet,* **2,** 876

14
Grain prolamins; why immunogenic, how toxic?

W.T.J.M. HEKKENS and M. VAN TWIST-DE GRAAF

Grain prolamins play a decisive role in the aetiology of coeliac disease. What is the special make-up of these prolamins to interfere with the intestinal lining in people with a genetic constitution that makes them sensitive to these molecules? This question implies the facts that the intestine of a normal individual does not react to the same prolamins and that no other proteins cause a similar damage to the intestinal wall in gluten-sensitive and in non-sensitive people.

THE NORMAL INTESTINE

Two of the main functions of the intestinal tract are of importance in relation to grain prolamins: the digestion of these proteins and the defense against unwanted or even toxic substances in the prolamins or formed from them during digestion. The normal intestinal lining is permeable for larger molecules, like proteins, not only in newborn babies, but also in adults. Walker[1] has studied this phenomenon and his conclusion is that up to about 10% of the proteins eaten can pass through the intestinal wall and trigger the immunological defense to react by the formation of antibodies and, at the same time, to develop a certain amount of tolerance to those alien molecules. In this general rule, prolamins are no exception. Antibodies against gliadin are found in the sera of premature and full-term babies as well as in adults. Normally the levels are low. In breastfed children, this level is the same as in children fed on cow's milk-based preparations. This phenomenon makes placental transmission of antibodies the most probable route. β-Lactoglobulin, one of the proteins from cow's milk, gives, in breastfed children, a similar pattern, whereas, in bottlefed children, the level of antibodies is increased, indicating that a second route of antigens must be open (Figure 1). Normally these antibodies reach a certain level and stay there for the rest of life. We determined the antigliadin antibodies in different age groups[2] and could demonstrate that, in adults, the level is

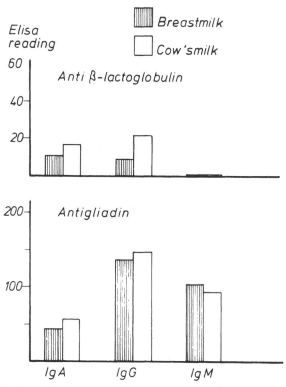

Figure 1 Antibodies against gliadin and β-lactoglobulin in premature babies on breastmilk or on cow's milk preparations

constant or even decreasing up to or over the age of 75 years (Figure 2). To the normal intestine, gliadin is certainly immunogenic; it is not toxic as we know from everyday life.

The immunological reaction is not the only reaction in the intestine. Studies by Troncone and Ferguson[3,4] have shown that gliadin is also a good tolerogen, at least in mice. Tolerance to proteins from food is one of the essential phenomena for survival. Differences in the development of tolerance could also be one of the causes of changes in reaction to different proteins and so play a role in the sensitivity to prolamins in coeliac patients.

The reaction to a substance depends not only on the concentration in which it is presented, but also on the duration. In the case of proteins in food, this means that the differences in rate of hydrolysis of the whole molecule, but also of the intermediate polypeptides, can be the cause of differences in immunogenicity or toxicity. It is well known that gliadin is one of the proteins that are only slowly digested. The rate of hydrolysis is greatly reduced in comparison with other food proteins[5].

THE AFFECTED INTESTINE

Fraser et al.[6] were the first to draw attention to the fact that digestion of gluten did not abolish toxicity for gluten-sensitive patients, starting a now

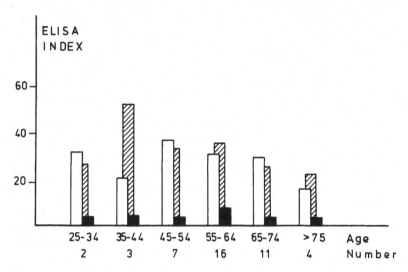

Figure 2 Antigliadin antibody levels in 43 healthy adults from different age groups. Black columns: IgA; white: IgG; hatched: IgM

thirty-year-long search for the peptide that must be responsible for the damage to the small intestine of coeliac patients.

Whether this damage is primarily caused by an immunological reaction or by a direct toxic effect is still not proven. The local cellular and antibody-mediated immune mechanism plays a pathogenic role as suggested by Bailey et al.[7]. This does not exclude, however, a direct effect of the (hydrophobic) peptides derived from gliadin on the permeability of the brush border membrane.

Davidson and Bridges[8] have carefully analysed the different hypotheses and conclude that none of them give a full explanation of the reactions observed after a gluten challenge. Although much is solved in the pathogenesis, the aetiology still remains obscure.

THE GRAIN PROLAMINS

The definition of prolamins, especially of wheat prolamins, goes back to 1907 when Osborne[9] published his thesis: *The Proteins of the Wheat Kernel*. Nearly all the work in the field of isolation is performed using his extraction methods. Attempts to make the solubility-based definition of gliadin more precise did not succeed. Electrophoresis has subdivided the gliadins into α-, β-, γ- and ω-gliadins[10], whereas two-dimensional electrophoresis has demonstrated that gliadin consists of about 50 different proteins[11]. Recent work based on peptide sequencing has indicated that the β-group is not an independent group but a mixture of a α-like and γ-like peptide sequences[12].

In 1970, we[13] published a study on the toxicity of a purified protein fraction isolated from that mixture of 50 proteins. We could prove the toxicity of the α-gliadin fraction and hoped that further purification could give us a single protein from which the structure could be established and the toxic peptide isolated.

In 1974, we[14] could prove that a peptide isolated from the tryptic digestion of that α-gliadin, with a molecular weight of about 18 000, was toxic to coeliac patients. The isolation of a sufficient amount of further purified and digested peptides became increasingly difficult and testing *in vivo* in patients is an ethical hazard.

In the meantime, Wieser *et al.*[15] had isolated a peptide starting from whole gliadin which turned out to be rather pure and which was toxic *in vitro* to biopsies taken from coeliac patients in the active phase. From this pure peptide of 54 amino acids, derived from the N-terminal side of gliadin, the sequence could be determined. They were able to isolate a pure peptide starting from such an impure material as gliadin because, in the different groups of gliadin, the N-terminal sequence is identical. This simplified the isolation substantially. The molecular weight of this peptide is approximately 6500, being about one third that of our peptide. As far as I know, this peptide has never been tested *in vivo*.

As Dicke, Weyers and van de Kamer[16] had already observed, the prolamins from rye and barley were also toxic to coeliac patients. To a lesser extent, oats are toxic too[17]. This makes it likely that these prolamins contain the same sequences as found in gliadin. In 1925, Lewis and Wells[18] compared the immunological properties of alcohol-soluble vegetable proteins. They found indeed that guinea pigs sensitized with wheat prolamins also had an anaphylactic shock when injected with the extracts from rye, barley and oats but not with extracts from maize.

The immunocrossreactivity means that there are shared epitopes in the different prolamins. One could wonder what these epitopes are and whether antigens against them have any relation to the toxic effect of the prolamins as experienced by gluten-sensitive patients.

When an antibody against gliadin is produced by a rabbit, this antibody will crossreact with prolamins isolated from other grains. Figure 3 demonstrates this crossreactivity. As can be seen, a crossreactivity with zein is also obtained with this rabbit antiserum. This means that a number of epitopes are shared by the different prolamins. As the antiserum is multivalent, more than one epitope is present. With a monoclonal antiserum, as shown by Ellis *et al.*[19], only a few bands are obtained. This demonstrates that the epitope reacting with the monoclonal antiserum is present in only two or three of the 50 proteins in gliadin. This leads to the conclusion that, in the proteins of the other prolamins, a number of bands sharing a number of different epitopes are made visible by antigliadin antiserum.

When we look at the amino acid sequences which can cause an antibody response when injected into a rabbit, we can see that a minimum of four amino acids at least is necessary. These four should preferably have a β-turn configuration. As shown in Table 1, from the work of Wieser *et al.*[12], it can be concluded that, in fact, there are many tetrapeptide sequences that are shared by the different prolamins to give rise to the great number of bands found in the immunocrossreactivity blots. The amount of pentapeptides is

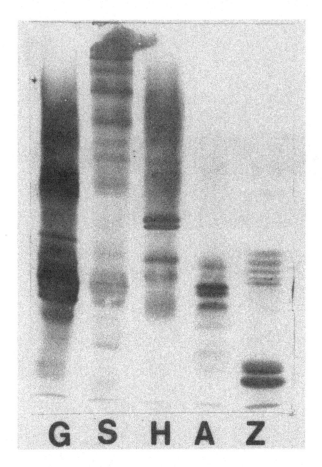

Figure 3 Immunocrossreactivity between the different prolamins and an antibody raised against gliadin. G, gliadin; S, secalin; H, hordein; A, avenin; Z, zein

much less and they are not shared in all the prolamins crossreacting with antigliadin. Moreover, from other analytical work by Tatham and his group[20], we know that about 35% of the α-gliadin chain is in the β-turn configuration. For the γ-chain, this amount is somewhat lower but still considerable. These β-turns are concentrated in the prolin-rich N-terminal repetitive domain and in the carboxy-terminal domain of the gliadin molecule.

One can imagine that the prolamins give rise to different amounts of antibodies, dependent of the number of epitopes presented to the antibody-producing cells. We, therefore, also raised antibodies against rye, barley, oats and zein to see whether there was a pattern of common bands in the prolamins from the different grains[21]. Figure 4 a–d gives the patterns obtained with the four antisera. From this, we can conclude that there is a number of bands shared by the first four prolamins. They do not, however, all have the same intensity. Bands that show intensive staining, with e.g.

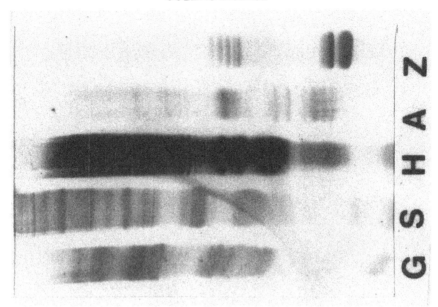

(b)

(a)

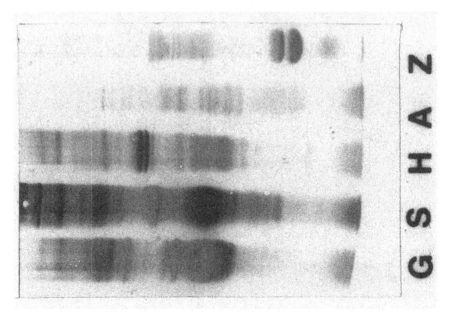

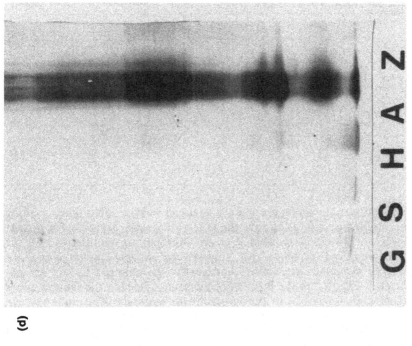

Figure 4 Immunocrossreactivity between the different prolamins and antibodies raised against: **a**, secalin; **b**, hordein; **c**, avenin and **d**, zein. Sequence of prolamins as in Figure 3

Table 1 Frequency of tetra- and pentapeptides in the repeating sequence domain of α-gliadin and hordein

Peptide	Number of residues	
	α-Gliadin	B-hordein
Gln.pro.phe.pro	3	5
Gln.gln.pro.phe	1	5
Pro.phe.pro.gln	1	4
Pro.tyr.pro.gln	2	3
Gln.pro.gln.pro	3	3
Gln.pro.tyr.pro	2	3
Gln.gln.pro.phe.pro	1	5
Gln.pro.phe.pro.gln	1	3
Gln.pro.tyr.pro.gln	2	3

antirye antiserum, can be found back as much weaker bands when reacting with antigliadin, indicating that the relative amounts are different or that exposure of B cells is reduced. For zein, the pattern is different. All the antisera we raised react with zein; however, the antizein antiserum does not react with the other prolamins. Apparently, the epitopes in zein are not sufficiently exposed to the B-cells to be immunogenic but the same epitopes in other grains give rise to the formation of antibody. This antibody can recognize the epitope in zein under the circumstances of the immunoblot. When we absorb the antisera with the different grains, the patterns obtained do not lead to a band or bands that are shared by all toxic grains, so the immunogenicity is not an unequivocal substitute for toxicity.

THE ANTIBODY PATTERN IN COELIAC DISEASE

Does gliadin induce a specific pattern of antibodies in patients that is not found in the serum of non-coeliac individuals?

Immunoblots of sera from patients with coeliac disease do not show a consistent pattern. They all have bands in the α-, β-, γ- and ω-regions of the gliadin in an immunoblot when the IgA, IgG or IgM antibodies are revealed. There are, however, many differences between patients on a normal diet. On a gluten-free diet over a sufficient period of time, all the bands return to the level found in normal individuals. Figure 5 illustrates some of these patterns. As far as we can see, there is no characteristic pattern in the immunoblots of patients with coeliac disease.

THE TOXIC LEVEL OF GLIADIN

To answer the question of the limit of toxicity is difficult. Ejderhamn et al.[22] have tried to establish the dose for which no effect on intestinal function or histology can be seen. They found that an amount of less than 13 mg per day over a period of 10 years did not produce any damage in 8 children of 15 years having coeliac disease.

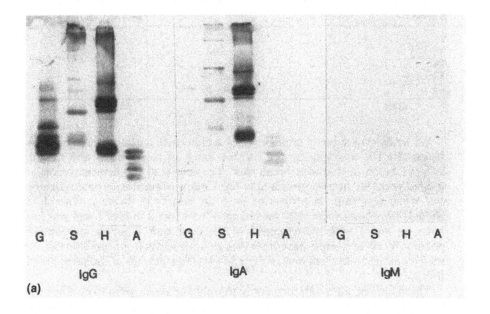

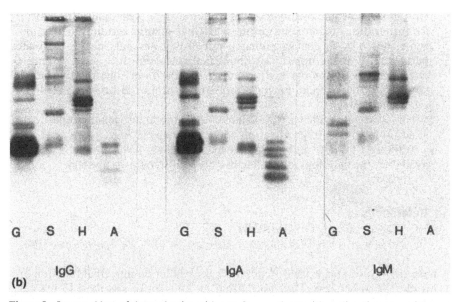

Figure 5 Immunoblots of the prolamins with sera from patients with coeliac disease. **a** with gluten-free diet; **b** no gluten-free diet

Table 2 ELISA analysis of different bread mixes used by a patient with coeliac disease

Sample	Batch	Gliadin (mg/100 g)
J	July '88	8
T	October '88	25
T1	July '88	3
T2	February '89	7
T3	February '89	3

We analysed the bread mixes used by a child with coeliac disease in order to explain the reaction she got on one batch of these mixes and not on another batch of the same bread mix. The results of the determination of gliadin with the method proposed to the Codex Alimentarius committee by our working group on prolamins gave the results in Table 2. The child showed symptoms soon after she changed from mix J to mix T and was put back on mix J with improvement of her condition. That the amount of gliadin in this mix must have been due to a difficulty in production can be seen from the analysis of one earlier and two later batches of the same bread mix.

These figures, although they apply to only one child, seem to confirm the conclusion of Ejderhamn that about 10 mg per day is the upper limit for a non-toxic effect.

CONCLUSION

On the basis of our own work over a period of 27 years and of the results from literature, the conclusion must be that gliadin certainly is immunogenic, not only in coeliac patients, but also in patients having a greater permeability of the upper gastrointestinal tract and, to a lesser extent, in normals. This immunogenicity stems from the poor digestibility and the structure of the protein, having a large proportion of β-turns in the N- and C-terminal region.

No clear-cut evidence is available that the tolerogenic properties of gliadin play a role in its effect on coeliac patients.

Although toxicity is better defined and levels have gradually become available, the aetiology of coeliac disease still remains a mystery.

References

1. Walker, W.A. (1982). Mechanisms of antigen handling by the gut. *Clin. Immunol. Allergy*, **2**, 15–40
2. Koot, C.V.M., van Straaten, M., Hekkens, W.Th.J.M., Collée, G. and Dijkmans, B.A.C. (1989). Elevated levels of IgA gliadin antibodies in patients with rheumatoid arthritis. *Clin. Exp. Rheum.* (in press)
3. Troncone, R. and Ferguson, A. (1988). Gliadin presented via the gut induces oral tolerance in mice. *Clin. Exp. Immunol.*, **72**, 284–287

4. Troncone, R. and Ferguson, A. (1988). In mice, gluten in maternal diet primes systemic immune responses to gliadin in offspring. *Immunology*, **64**, 533–537
5. Zimmerman-Nielsen, C. and Schonheyder, F. (1962). On the rate of disappearance of protein from the small intestine in vivo. *Biochim. Biophys. Acta*, **63**, 201–203
6. Frazer, A.C., Fletcher, R.F., Shaw, B., Ross, C.A.C., Sammons, G.H. and Schneider, R. (1959). Gluten-induced enteropathy. The effect of partially digested gluten. *Lancet*, **2**, 252–255
7. Baily, D.S., Freedman, A.R., Price, S.C., Chescoe, D. and Ciclitira, P.J. (1989). Early biochemical responses of the small intestine of coeliac patients to wheat gluten. *Gut*, **30**, 78–85
8. Davidson, A.G.F. and Bridges, M.A. (1987). Coeliac disease: a critical review of aetiology and pathogenesis. *Clin. Chim. Acta*, **163**, 1–40
9. Osborne, T.B. (1907). The proteins of the wheat kernel. *Thesis*, Carnegie Institute (Washington Publ. 84)
10. Jones, R.W., Taylor, N.W. and Senti, F.R. (1959). Electrophoresis and fractionation of wheat gluten. *Arch. Biochem.*, **84**, 363–376
11. Wrigley, C.W. and Shephard, K.W. (1973). Electrofocussing of grain proteins from wheat genotypes. *Ann. N.Y. Acad. Sci.*, **209**, 154
12. Wieser, H., Seilmeier, W. and Belitz, H.D. (1987). Vergleichende Untersuchungen über partiëlle Aminosäuresequenzen von Prolaminen und Glutelinen verschiedener Getreidearten. *Z. Lebensm. Unters. Forsch.*, **184**, 366–373
13. Hekkens, W.Th.J.M., Haex, A.J.Ch. and Willighagen, R.G.J. (1970). Some aspects of gliadin fractionation and testing by a histochemical method. In Booth, C.C. and Dowling, R.H. (eds.) *Coeliac Disease. Proceedings International Coeliac Symposium*, pp. 11–19 (Edinburgh: Churchill Livingstone)
14. Hekkens, W.Th.J.M., van den Aarsen, C.J., Gilliams, J.P., Lems-van Kan, Ph. and Bouma-Frölich, G. (1974). α-Gliadin structure and degradation. In Hekkens, W.Th.J.M. and Pena, A.S. (eds.) *Coeliac Disease. Proceedings Second International Coeliac Symposium*, pp. 39–45. (Leiden: Stenfert Kroese)
15. Wieser, H., Belitz, H.D. and Ashkenazi, A. (1984). Amino-acid sequence of the coeliac active gliadin peptide B3142. *Z. Lebensm. Unters. Forsch.*, **179**, 371–376
16. Dicke, W.K., Weyers, H.A. and van de Kamer, J.H. (1953). Coeliac disease II. The presence in wheat of a factor having a deleterious effect in cases of coeliac disease. *Acta Paediatr.*, **42**, 34–42
17. Hansted, C.A.E. (1956). Results of investigations concerning food with harmful effect ("gluten-effect") on patients with coeliac disease. In *8th International Congress of Paediatrics*, Copenhagen. *Acta Paediatr.*, **45**, E137
18. Lewis, J.H. and Wells, H.G. (1925). The immunological properties of alcohol-soluble vegetable proteins. *J. Biol. Chem.*, **66**, 37–48
19. Ellis, H.J., Freedman, A.R. and Ciclitira, P.J. (1989). The production and characterisation of monoclonal antibodies to wheat gliadin peptides. *J. Immun. Meth.*, **120**, 17–22
20. Tatham, A.S., Miflin, B.J. and Shewry, P.R. (1985). The beta-turn conformation in wheat gluten proteins: Relationship to gluten elasticity. *Cereal Chem.*, **62**, 405–412
21. van Twist-de Graaf, M.J., Wieser, H. and Hekkens, W.Th.J.M. (1989). Immunocrossreactivity of antisera against grain prolamins of wheat, rye, barley and oats. *Z. Lebensm. Unters. Forsch.*, **188**, 535–539
22. Ejderhamn, J., Veress, B. and Strandvik, B. (1988). The long term effect of continual ingestion of wheat starch containing gluten-free products in celiac patients. In *Proceedings Fourth International Symposium on Coeliac Disease*, London 1988, in press

15
Class II molecules in coeliac disease

M.L. MEARIN

Genetic immunological and environmental factors are necessary for the clinical expression of coeliac disease (CD). For many years, CD has been considered to be a familial disorder because it was known that some families could have several coeliac members[1-3]. The role of genetic factors has been substantiated by the high concordance rate in monozygotic twins[4] (70%) as compared with dizygotic twins (30%).

THE HLA-COMPLEX

In 1972, two different groups of investigators[5,6] found an association between CD and the histocompatibility antigen, HLA-B8. The HLA specificities are cell membrane antigens coded by the major histocompatibility complex genes (the HLA-complex) situated in the short arm of chromosome 6. The HLA-complex genes are divided into 3 categories: class I, II and III (Figure 1). Each class II gene locus has a gene for an α and β subunit of a class II antigen and both of these genes may express polymorphism. The HLA-complex genes class I and II have several loci (class I: HLA-A, -B and -C; class II: HLA-DR, -DQ, -DO, -DZ and -DP); the loci have several alleles. The individual HLA specificities are inherited as codominant alleles: for each locus, two gene products can be detected unless there is homozygosity for one antigen. The combination of antigens determined by one HLA chromosomal region is inherited as a unit: the HLA-haplotype. It is characteristic of the HLA polymorphism that some haplotype frequencies in the population are greater than would be expected from the products of the individual gene frequencies. These allelic associations are named linkage desequilibrium and are often quite marked (e.g. HLA-A1, -B8, -DR3; HLA-A3 and -B7). It is thought that, if a disease susceptibility gene were to exist in the HLA chromosomal region, it would also hitch-hike with the selected gene and with closely linked alleles in this region[7].

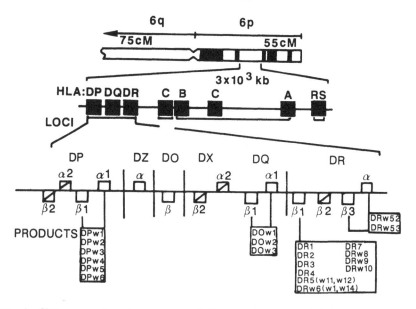

Figure 1 Chromosome 6, major histocompatibility complex genes and their products

THE HLA-CLASS II MOLECULES

Even though the first association between CD and the HLA system[5,6] was found with the HLA-class I molecules -A1 and -B8, shortly thereafter, it was shown[8] that CD has a stronger association with the HLA-class II molecule -DW3; the association with class I molecules was found to be due to linkage desequilibrium.

MHC class II molecules have a role in the immune response by presenting antigens to the T cell receptors and most diseases showing association with HLA do associate with class II molecules. However, the underlying mechanisms which account for this relationship are not well understood. Several mechanisms have been proposed, such as the HLA antigens serving as surface receptors for viruses or toxic substances, or the molecular mimicry of the HLA-molecules with the chemical structure of these substances allowing them to appear as self antigens[9]. It is reasonable that the antigen-presenting capacity of a particular combination of class II molecules determines whether immunological responses to a toxic substance are possible on a genetic level.

Population studies in different countries have confirmed the association of CD with the HLA class II molecules, HLA-DR3 and -DR7, and with the HLA-DR phenotypes, DR3/DR7[10-14], DR3/DR3[13,14] and DR5/DR7[13]. Large-scale family studies have also shown that CD segregates with these HLA-DR phenotypes[12-14] (Table 1). In studies on Spanish and Dutch children with CD[13,14], it was found that 98% of the patients had at least one of the HLA-DR antigens -DR3, -DR5 or -DR7. Among the Dutch children with CD, all had at least one of the antigens -DR3, -DR7, -DR4 or -DR5. In

Table 1 Segregation of coeliac disease with certain HLA-DR phenotypes in family studies

Parents	Phenotype	Coeliac children	Healthy siblings
One parent	DR3/DR7	9	6
heterozygous for	DR3/-	3	10
DR3 and the	DR7/-	2	3
other for DR7	-/-	0	10
		(n = 14)	(n = 29)
One parent	DR7/DR5	4	1
heterozygous for	DR7/+	1	1
DR7 and the	DR5/+	0	2
other for DR5	+/+	0	2
		(n = 5)	(n = 6)
Both parents	DR3/DR3	6	3
heterozygous	3/#	5	3
for DR3	#/#	0	4
		(n = 11)	(n = 10)

From reference 13. – = another antigen different from DR3 or DR7; + = another antigen different from DR7 or DR5; # = another antigen different from DR3

both studies, the HLA-phenotypes lacking HLA-DR3, -DR4, -DR5 or -DR7 had a highly significant negative association with CD.

In 1983, Tosi et al.[15] described, among HLA-DR3-DR7-positive coeliac patients, a 100% association of the disease with the HLA class II molecule, DQw2, which is in linkage disequilibrium with HLA-DR3 and -DR7. At that point, the association of CD with the haplotype, HLA-DR7/DR5, was not well understood. Later investigations have shown that HLA-DR3-DR7-negative coeliac patients are not always HLA-DQw2 positive, but are DR4 positive[16].

One of the respects in which HLA-DQ molecules differ from HLA-DR ones is that both the α and the β chain genes are polymorphic in the HLA-DQ; polymorphism of the HLA-DR molecules is limited to the β chains[17]. This is the reason why hybrid HLA-DQ molecules can result from gene transcomplementation in heterozygous cells for DQα and/or DQβ. Bontrop et al.[18], using electrophoretic analysis of immunoprecipitated HLA-DQ molecules, found five different HLA-DQ α- and six HLA-DQ β-chain gene products, indicating that 30 different HLA-DQα/β dimers theoretically can occur. In fact, within a panel of 29 HLA-DR-DQ homozygous B-cell lines, only 10 DQα/β dimers could be identified.

The HLA-DQw2 allospecificity is associated with 2 types of α/β dimers: DQ α2.3/β1.2 and with DQα2.7/β2.7. On the other hand, the same type of DQα or DQβ chains can be expressed by cell lines with different HLA-DR-DQ haplotypes. For example, the HLA-DQα2.3 chain can be expressed by cell lines with the haplotype DR3-Dw3-DQw2 as well as by cell lines with haplotype DR4-Dw4-DQw3. Thus, it is possible that the same HLA-DRα/β dimers are coded by different HLA-DR-DQ haplotypes.

In 1988, Roep et al.[19] showed, at both the DNA and protein levels, that CD is strongly associated with the HLA-DQ chains α2.3, β2.7, and, to a lesser extent, with the HLA-DQβ2.3 chain. From 2D gel analysis, they suggested that, at the cell surface, HLA-DQα2.3 probably associates with the HLA-DQβ2.7 or HLA-DQβ2.3 chain. In some cases, this association may be the result of transcomplementation; for example, the maternal haplotype may bring in the HLA-DQα2.3 whereas the paternal haplotype codes for the HLA-DQβ2.7 or HLA-DQβ2.3. Roep *et al.* speculated that the HLA-DQα2.3/HLA-DQβ2.7 dimer, or, to a lesser extent, the HLA-DQα2.3/HLA-DQβ2.3 dimer, are the putative HLA class II molecules involved in the onset of CD. Recently, Sollid *et al.*[20] have shown that 93 of 94 unrelated children with CD may share a particular HLA-DQα/β heterodimer encoded by the combination of two HLA-DQ genes (HLA-DQA1 and DQB1). These genes are arranged in *cis* position on the DR3DQw2 haplotype and in *trans* position in DR5DQw7/DR7DQw2 heterozygous individuals. Their findings have greatly helped to explain why CD is associated with different HLA-DR-DQ haplotypes. DNA analysis had already revealed almost identical nucleotide sequences of the DR3DQw2 and DR5Dw7 haplotypes of the DQA1 genes and of the DR3DQw2 and DR7DQw2 haplotypes of the DQB1 genes[21], indicating a common origin of these genes. Thus, the genetic information of the DR3DQw2 haplotype is re-established in DR5DQw7/DR7DQw2 heterozygotes though the genes are split between two chromosomes. It was known too[22] that the amino acid sequence of the DQβ chain encoded by the DR3DQw2 haplotype is identical to that encoded by the DR5DQw7, while the DQ chain of the DR3DQw2 haplotype is identical to that of the DR7DQw2 except for a single amino acid difference in the second domain.

In their studies at DNA level, Sollid *et al.*[20] found that probes of the DQA1 and DQB1 genes hybridized to DNA from 93 out of 94 CD patients in comparison with 14 out of 56 healthy controls. The only CD patient whose DNA did not hybridize to the DQA1 and DQB1 probes was DR4w6. Thus, most of CD patients may share a particular combination of DQA1 and DQB1 genes and it is possible that, by transcomplementation, a coeliac patient who is DR5Qw7/DR7DQw2 may express the same DQα/β heterodimer as the one encoded by the DQA1 and DQB1 genes in *cis* position on the DR3DQw2 haplotype.

Apart from the association between CD and the DR- and DQ- genes, other reports have indicated an association between CD and some DP polymorphisms[23]. Whether all those genes contribute to susceptibility for CD or whether their associations are secondary to the one with DQ is not yet known.

THE HLA-II MOLECULES AND THE SMALL INTESTINE

The mucosa of the small intestine of patients with CD is the target organ of the pathological mechanisms triggered by gliadin. According to the immunological theory for the aetiology of CD, it is tempting to speculate that the central defect resides in the abnormal immune response to gliadin mounted by the mucosa of the small intestine because of the presence of specific HLA class II molecules. Several studies on the subject have shown different patterns of HLA class II-molecule expressions at small intestine level in CD.

Scott et al.[24] were the first to report the expression of HLA-DR on normal villous epithelium in an apical granular distribution. More studies show increased expression of HLA-DR, both in surface and crypt epithelium as well as in lamina propria lymphocytes of untreated CD patients[25-27]. This increased epithelial class II expression is thought to be related to immunological activity in the mucosa of CD patients.

In their studies with frozen sections of jejunal mucosa from treated and untreated coeliac patients, Marley et al.[27] found a pattern of DR > DP > DQ staining using monoclonal antibodies to the different class II antigenic specificities subgroups. The staining was observed most strongly in the villous enterocytes and decreased towards the crypt bases. Kelly et al.[28], in their studies on the differential expression of HLA-D gene products in normal and coeliac small bowel using monoclonal antibodies, found that the HLA-DQ antigens showed a similar distribution, being absent from epithelial cells and present only in cells within the lamina propria. Schweizer et al.[29], using specific monoclonal antibodies to the HLA-DQα2.3 and HLA-DQβ2.7 chains (which are highly associated to CD), have found that those chains are expressed in the lamina propria of the small intestine in both CD patients and HLA-matched controls (Figure 2). No expression of the HLA-DQα2.3 or of the HLA-DQβ2.7 was found in the enterocytes of either group. Recently, Bonamico et al.[30] did not find HLA-DQ expression on the enterocytes of coeliac patients but did show statistically significant differences in expression of DP antigens on enterocytes of coelic patients on gluten-containing diet or after gluten challenge in comparison with coeliac patients on a gluten-free diet or with controls.

Two possible roles for class II molecules in the small intestinal epithelium have been proposed[31]. First, the enterocyte may be directly involved in antigen presentation. Second, enterocyte class II molecules may act as binding antigen molecules. If that is the case, it does not seem probable that the HLA-DQ heterodimers would be involved in the presentation of gliadin peptides in CD. It is more likely that the HLA-DQα/β dimers have a regulatory function in the immune response to gliadin once it has crossed the small intestine epithelium.

References

1. MacDonald, W.C., Dobbins, W.D. and Rubin, C.E. (1965). Studies on the familial nature of celiac sprue using biopsy of the small intestine. N. Engl. J. Med., 272, 448–456
2. Robinson, D.C., Watson, A.J., Wyatt, E.H., Marks, J.M. and Roberts, D.F. (1971). Incidence of small-intestinal mucosa abnormalities and of clinical coeliac disease in the relatives of children with coeliac disease. Gut, 12, 189–193
3. Rolles, C.J., Kyaw-Myint, T.B., Sin, K.W. and Anderson, Ch.M. (1981). The familial incidence of asymptomatic coeliac disease. In McConell, R.B. (ed.) The Genetics of Coeliac Disease, pp. 235–250. (Lancaster: MTP Press)
4. Peña, A.S. (1982). Genetics of coeliac disease. In Jewell, D.P. and Lee, E. (eds.) Topics in Gastroenterology, pp. 62–81. (Oxford: Blackwell)
5. Stokes, P.L., Asquith, P., Holmes, G.K.T., MacKintosch, P. and Cooke, W.T. (1972). Histocompatibility antigens associated with adult coeliac disease. Lancet, 2, 162–164
6. Falchuck, Z.M., Rogentine, G.N. and Strober, W. (1972). Predominance of histocompatibility antigen HLA8 in patients with gluten-sensitive enteropathy. J. Clin. Invest., 51, 1602–1605

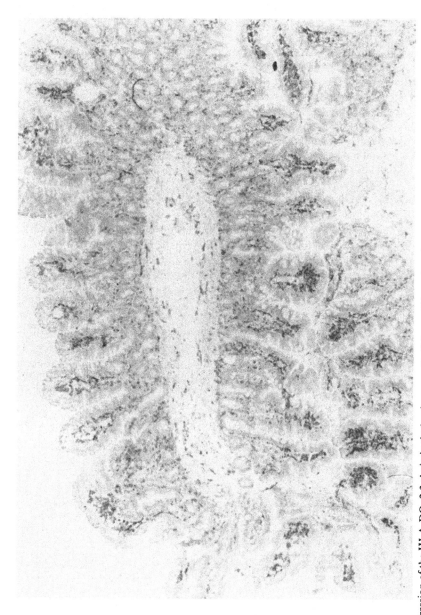

Figure 2 Expression of the HLA-DQα2.3 chain in the lamina propria of the small intestine of a coeliac patient using an immunoperoxidase technique and the monoclonal antibody SFR20-Dα5. From reference 29

7. Woodrow, J.C. (1981). The HLA-system. In McConell, R.B. (ed.) *The Genetics of Coeliac Disease*, pp. 111–121. (Lancaster: MTP Press)

8. Keuning, J.J., Peña, A.S., van Leeuwen, A., van Hoof, J.P. and van Rood, J.J. (1976). HLA-Dw3 associated with coeliac disease. *Lancet*, 1, 506–507

9. Strober, W. (1981). The influence of histocompatibility genes on the pathogenesis of gluten sensitive enteropathy. In McConell, R.B. (ed.) *The Genetics of Coeliac Disease*, pp. 183–193. (Lancaster: MTP Press)

10. De Marchi, M., Borelli, Y., Olivetti, E., Richardi, P., Wright, C., Ansaldi, N., Barbera, C. and Santini, B. (1979). Two HLA-D and DR alleles are associated with coeliac disease. *Tiss. Antigens*, 14, 309–316

11. Betuel, H., Gebuhrer, L., Descos, L., Percebois, H., Minaire, Y. and Bertrand, J. (1980). Adult celiac disease associated with HLA-DRw3 and -DRw7. *Tiss. Antigens*, 15, 231–242

12. Brautbar, C., Freier, S., Ashkenazi, A., Dekelbaum, R., Tur-Kasper, I., Amar, A., Cohen, I., Sharon, R., Abecassis, R., Levine, C., Cohen, T. and Albert, E. (1981). Histocompatibility determinants in Israeli Jewish patients with coeliac disease: population and family study. *Tiss. Antigens*, 17, 313–322

13. Mearin, M.L., Biemond, I., Peña, A.S., Polanco, I., Vazquez, C., Schreuder, G.Th.M., de Vries, R.R.P. and van Rood, J.J. (1983). HLA-DR phenotypes in Spanish coeliac children: their contribution to the understanding of the genetics of the disease. *Gut*, 24, 532–537

14. Mearin, M.L., Bouquet, I., Mourad, N., Schoorel, E., Sinaasappel, M., Biemond, I., Schreuder, A.Th.M., Peña, A.S., van Gelderen, H.H. and van Rood, J.J. (1985). HLA-DR antigens and phenotypes in Dutch coeliac children and their families. *Clin. Gen.*, 27, 45–50

15. Tosi, R., Vismara, D., Tanigaki, N., Ferrara, G.B., Cicimarra, F., Boffalano, W., Follo, D. and Aurichio, S. (1983). Evidence that celiac disease is primarily associated with a DC locus allelic specificity. *Clin. Immunol. Immunopathol.*, 28, 395–404

16. Tosi, R., Tanigaki, N., Polanco, I., De Marchi, M., Woodrow, S.C. and Hetzel, Ph.A. (1986). A radioimmunoassay typing study of non DQw2 associated coeliac disease. *Clin. Immunol. Immunopathol.*, 39, 168–172

17. Schenning, L., Larhammar, D., Bill, P., Wiman, K., Johsson, A., Rask, L. and Peterson, P.A. (1984). Both α and β chains of HLA-DC class II histocompatibility antigens display extensive polymorphism in their amino terminal domains. *EMBO J.*, 3, 447–452

18. Bontrop, R.E., Baas, E.J., Otting, N., Schreuder, G.H.T. and Giphart, M.J. (1987). Molecular diversity of HLA-DQ. DQ-alpha and -beta chain isoelectric point differences and their relation to serologically defined HLA-DQ allospecificities. *Immunogenetics*, 25, 305–312

19. Roep, B.O., Bontrop, R.E., Peña, A.S., van Eggermond, M.C.J.A., van Rood, J.J. and Giphart, M.J. (1988). An HLA-DQ alpha allele identified at DNA and protein level is strongly associated with coeliac disease. *Hum. Immunol.*, 23, 271–279

20. Sollid, L.M., Markussen, G., Ek, J., Gjerde, H., Vartdal, F. and Thorsby, E. (1989). Evidence for a primary association of celiac disease to a particular HLA-DQα/β heterodimer. *J. Exp. Med.*, 169, 345–350

21. Karr, R.W., Gregersen, P.K., Obata, F., Goldberg, D., Maccari, J., Alber, C. and Silver, J. (1986). Analysis of DRβ and DQβ chain cDNA clones from a DR7 haplotype. *J. Immunol.*, 137, 2886–2890

22. Schiffenbauer, J., Didier, D.K., Klearman, M., Rice, K., Shuman, S., Tieber, V.L., Kittlesen, D.J. and Schwartz, B.D. (1987). Complete sequence of the HLA DQα and DQβ cDNA from a DR5/DQw3 cell line. *J. Immunol.*, 139, 228–233

23. Niven, M.J., Caffrey, J.C., Sachs, J.A., Cassell, P.G., Gallagher, R.B., Kumar, P. and Hitman, G.A. (1987). Susceptibility to coeliac disease involves genes in HLA-DP region. *Lancet*, 2, 805

24. Scott, H., Solheim, B.G., Brandtzaeg, P. and Thorsby, E. (1981). HLA-DR like antigens in the epithelium of the human small intestine. *Scand. J. Immunol.*, 12, 77–82

25. Arnaud Batandier, F., Cerf-Bensussan, N., Amsellem, R. and Schmitz, J. (1986). Increased HLA-DR expression by enterocytes in children with coeliac disease. *Gastroenterology*, 91, 1205–1212

26. Ciclitira, P.J., Nuluger, S.M., Ellis, H.J. and Evans, D.J. (1986). The effect of gluten on HLA-DR in the small intestinal epithelium of patients with coeliac disease. *Clin. Exp. Immunol.*, 63, 101–104

27. Marley, N.J.E., Macarthey, J.C. and Ciclitira, P.J. (1987). HLA-DR, DP and DQ

expression in the small intestine of patients with coeliac disease. *Clin. Exp. Immunol.,* **70,** 386–393

28. Kelly, J., Weir, D.G. and Faighery, C. (1988). Differential expression of HLA-D gene products in the normal and coeliac small bowel. *Tiss. Antigens,* **29,** 151–160

29. Schweizer, J.J., Mearin, M.L., Peña, A.S., Offerhaus, G.J.A., Dreef, E.J., Roep, B.O., Bontrop, R.E., Dooren, L.J., Lamers, C.B.H.W. and Hoedemaeker, Ph.J. (1990). HLA-DQ specific alleles strongly associated with coeliac disease are expressed at the small intestinal level in patients suffering from coeliac disease and in HLA-matched controls. *In preparation*

30. Bonamico, M., Mazzilli, M.C., Morellini, M., Vania, A., Carpino, F., Nicotra, M.R. and Natili, P.G. (1989). Expression of class II MHC antigens in the intestinal epithelium of pediatric celiac disease. *J. Paediatr. Gastroenterol. Nutr.,* **9,** 269–275

31. Bland, P. (1988). MHC class II expression by the gut epithelium. *Immunol. Today,* **9,** 174–178

16
The diagnostic significance of gliadin and endomysium antibodies in childhood coeliac disease

A. BÜRGIN-WOLFF, H. GAZE, F. HADZISELIMOVIC, M.J. LENTZE and D. NUSSLÉ

INTRODUCTION

It is well known that the formation of small amounts of antibodies (ab) to ingested proteins is a normal physiological occurrence. Low levels of antibodies to proteins in nutrients can therefore be demonstrated in nearly all persons, provided the test method used is sensitive enough. This is also true for antibodies against gliadin (AGA).

In 1958, it was first shown by E. Berger in the Basle Children's hospital that elevated quantities of antibodies to gliadin were associated with gluten enteropathy[1]. We subsequently tried to establish a simple and reliable test for measuring gliadin ab in different immunoglobulin classes[2]. This test was expected to be useful for diagnostic purposes[3-6]. The aim was, therefore, to discriminate between coeliac patients and patients with other malabsorptive disorders, and not to detect the very low levels of antibody physiologically present in nearly all healthy individuals.

In the last few years, several papers have appeared on the determination of antibodies against gliadin as a screening test for coeliac disease (CD). Most authors agree that IgG antibody determinations are sensitive but not pathognomonic while IgA ab are more specific but are less sensitive[7-17].

In 1983, Chorzelsky et al. described antibodies against endomysium and found a close correlation between these ab and patients with dermatitis herpetiformis[18]. Later on, they also found endomysium ab in coeliac patients[19]. Endomysium ab are directed against extracellular reticular fibres in the endomysium that surrounds the smooth muscle cells of many species.

Our aim was now to compare the diagnostic significance of gliadin ab with endomysium ab in patients with untreated CD, in disease controls, in patients with CD on a gliadin-free diet, and after reintroduction of gluten into the food.

PATIENTS

We included in this study:

(1) 656 patients, who had undergone a first jejunal biopsy because of suspected CD, from children's hospitals throughout Switzerland and the Federal Republic of Germany. Their ages ranged from 2 months to 18 years (mean age 2.7 years). All were under investigation for gastrointestinal disease, failure to thrive, iron deficiency anaemia, short stature and other malabsorptive disorders. At the time of blood sampling, they were all on a gliadin-containing diet.

(2) 86 children, with multiple blood samples, on a gliadin-free diet for varying periods.

(3) 124 patients with morphological relapse after reintroduction of gliadin into the diet.

(4) Coeliac patients without relapse.

At the time of gliadin ab determinations, the biopsy results were not known. Endomysium ab determinations were often performed retrospectively in the serum samples still available.

METHODS

Determination of gliadin ab

The fluorescent immunosorbent test (FIST) was used for the determination of ab against gliadin as described elsewhere[2,3,5].

Determination of endomysium ab

Unfixed cryostat sections of monkey oesophagus were incubated with the patients' serum, mostly diluted 1:10 in PBS. They are made visible by overlying the sections with a fluorescent anti-IgA serum in an appropriate dilution. Under the fluorescence microscope, a brilliant green network is seen, especially in the lamina muscularis.

Statistical evaluation

The methods used for statistical evaluation of gliadin ab are described elsewhere[5].

Table 1 IgG and IgA antibodies to gliadin compared with biopsy findings (*n* = 656)

	Untreated CD, flat mucosa (mean age 1.8 years) (n = 392)	Disease controls, normal mucosa or partial villous atrophy (mean age 3.5 years) (n = 264)
IgG and IgA ab positive	347 (89%)	10 (4%)
Only IgG ab positive		
high titre	31 (8%)	16 (6%)
low titre	12 (3%)	28 (11%)
Only IgA ab positive	0 (0%)	0 (0%)
No antibodies	2 (0.5%)	210 (80%)

RESULTS

Antibodies in children with untreated CD and in controls

IgG and IgA gliadin antibodies

In Table 1, the results of gliadin ab determinations are compared with the histological findings in the intestinal mucosae of 656 children with jejunal biopsy. Of the 392 children with a flat mucosa, 390 (99.5%) had IgG ab, and 347 of them (89%) also had IgA ab. In only two patients, no ab could be found. One of them was a 6-year-old boy with short stature and a selective total IgA deficiency; the other was a three-year-old girl.

On the other hand, 80% of the 264 controls with a normal or only slightly pathological mucosa had neither IgG nor IgA gliadin ab. IgG ab were present in 17%, most of them in low titres, whereas only 4% had IgG and IgA ab to gliadin. Children never had IgA gliadin ab alone. Most coeliac patients had high ab titres, although the titres tend to decline with age[5].

The above data show that, for diagnostic purposes, neither solely IgG nor solely IgA AGA determinations give satisfactory results. The combined results, however, are well suited as a screening test for coeliac disease. Although the methods for determining gliadin ab are not yet standardized, the Italian group of Guandalini recently presented exactly the same results[20] in a very large study.

IgE gliadin antibodies

Very little is known about IgE-class ab in coeliac disease. In our study, 92% of children with a flat mucosa had IgE gliadin ab. However, 21.5% of children with a normal mucosa or partial villous atrophy also produced IgE ab (Table 2). Therefore, these antibodies are less reliable indicators of CD than IgA-ab (for details see reference 5).

The pathogenetic role of different immunoglobulin classes of gliadin-ab is unknown.

Table 2 IgE antibodies to gliadin compared with biopsy findings, $n = 294$

	IgE ab positive/total
Untreated CD	163/178 (92%)
Disease controls	25/116 (22%)

Endomysium ab (EMA)

Of 337 patients with *untreated* CD, 90% had ab to endomysium (Table 3). Their frequency was roughly the same in patients with and without IgA gliadin ab. In fact, one of the two children without any gliadin ab produced endomysium ab. On the other hand (Table 4), we found EMA in only 4/211 disease controls. Ninety-eight per cent of the patients with a normal mucosa or only partial villous atrophy were negative. The endomysium ab test is therefore very specific for CD but not as sensitive as gliadin ab determination. The sensitivity of the endomysium ab test is 90% compared with at least 96% with gliadin ab determination[5]. It is interesting that the false negative patients are all younger than two years old. We do not know, at present, whether some of them are children with transient gluten intolerance.

Table 3 IgG and IgA ab to gliadin and endomysium, *untreated CD* (flat mucosa), $n = 337$

	Endomysium ab	
Gliadin ab	Positive 304/337 (90%)	Negative 33/337 (10%)
IgA and IgG ab positive, $n = 271$	247	24
Only IgG ab positive, $n = 64$	56	8
No antibodies, $n = 2$	1	1

Table 4 IgG and IgA ab to gliadin and endomysium, *no coeliac disease, $n = 211$* (normal mucosa or partial villous atrophy)

	Endomysium ab	
Gliadin ab	Positive 4/211 (2%)	Negative 207/211 (98%)
IgA and IgG ab positive, $n = 12$	1	11
Only IgG ab positive, $n = 62$	2	60
No antibodies, $n = 137$	1	136

Antibodies in children on a gluten-free diet

Gliadin antibodies, like endomysium ab, disappear under a gluten-free diet. IgA gliadin ab disappear very quickly (2–6 months) so that they are useful as a diet control. By contrast, IgG gliadin ab need a long time, sometimes more than a year to become negative. As an example the time course of the corresponding antibody titres in 11 patients on a gluten-free diet is shown in Figure 1. Endomysium ab persist longer than IgA gliadin ab but not as long as IgG gliadin ab. Figure 2 shows the percentages of sera that are still positive in 86 patients with multiple blood samples after increasing periods on a gluten-free diet.

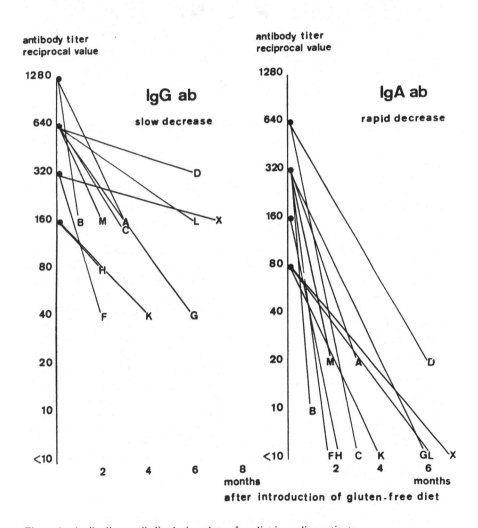

Figure 1   Antibodies to gliadin during gluten-free diet in coeliac patients

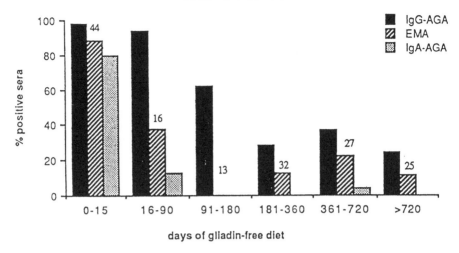

Figure 2   Frequency of antibodies to gliadin and endomysium during gliadin-free diet

Antibodies in children after reintroduction of gluten into the diet

Gliadin ab

To demonstrate the persistence of gluten intolerance, coeliac patients are often challenged with gluten. IgG, as well as IgA gliadin ab, are, in general, produced shortly after the beginning of the challenge as shown in Figure 3. Thirty-six out of 40 patients with a morphological relapse at the end of the challenge period had increasing ab titres within 4 weeks. Four of the antibody-positive patients still had a normal mucosa at that time (open circles in Figure 4). One patient did not produce any gliadin ab although he showed a damaged mucosa after 9 months of challenge.

If a normal gluten-containing diet is reintroduced in coeliac patients for long periods, the following may happen: in the initial phase the *gliadin-ab titres* increase but later on they may decline again and, in some patients, even become negative, although the biopsy shows a severely damaged mucosa at the end of the challenge (Figure 4). An unwanted challenge of this kind sometimes happens in paediatric treatment, namely when patients do not keep to their diet and are biopsied after some years of 'sins'. If, in these patients, the gliadin ab were tested only once at the end of the long period of challenge, the initial ab increase would go unnoticed because the serological result would be negative in spite of a pathological mucosa. It is important to see that a negative gliadin ab titre does not rule out a persistent gluten intolerance in this kind of patient.

Endomysium ab

Endomysium ab are produced later in challenge than gliadin ab but they do not disappear after a prolonged challenge (Figure 5). The percentage of sera with gliadin ab is highest (96%) after a challenge period of about 4 weeks to

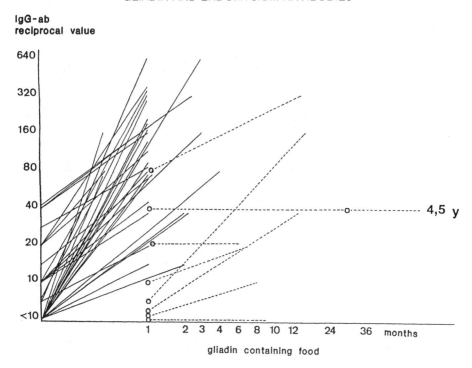

Figure 3   IgG gliadin-ab before and after challenge in coeliac disease ($n = 40$). ──── mucosa normal before and pathological after 1 month of challenge ($n = 32$); O – – – mucosa normal after 1 month of challenge, pathological after prolonged challenge ($n = 8$)

3 months and afterwards decreases to about 50% after 3 or more years of gliadin intake. By contrast, the percentage of endomysium-ab-positive patients is highest after one year on normal food and stays at that level even after very long periods of gliadin intake.

SUMMARY AND COMMENTS

Ab determination as a screening test for untreated CD in childhood

Table 5 summarizes the results of gliadin and endomysium ab determinations. It is obvious that the combined determination of these ab gives an excellent prediction of the condition of the mucosa, particularly in all those patients with three concordant ab results. It takes advantage of the very high sensitivity of gliadin ab determination and the very high specificity of endomysium ab determination.

Of the 248 patients with three *positive* tests, namely positive EMA and positive IgA as well as positive IgG gliadin ab, 247 or 99.6% had a flat mucosa and were therefore serologically correctly diagnosed. Only one showed a normal mucosa. The percentage of patients with flat mucosae decreases if only one or two tests are positive. On the other hand, 136 out of

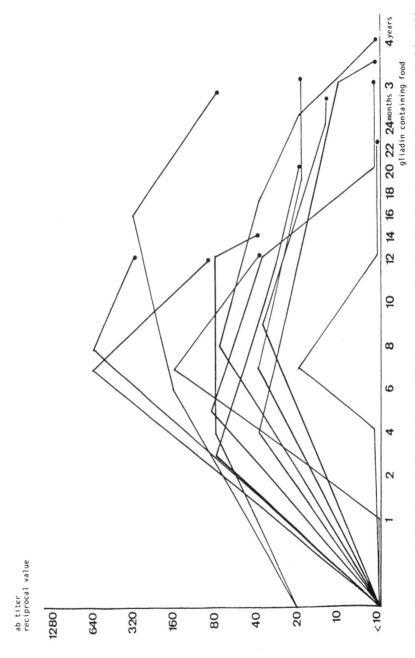

Figure 4 IgG antibodies to gliadin before and after gliadin-containing food over a prolonged period. 12 patients with relapse proven by jejunal biopsy at the end of the observation period ●

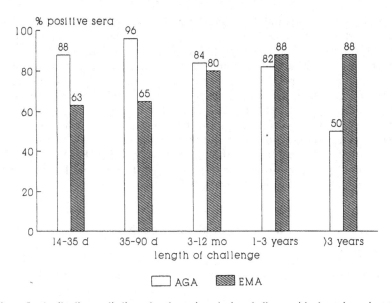

Figure 5 Antibodies to gliadin and endomysium during challenge with gluten in patients with relapse. 274 sera of 93 patients

Table 5 Antibodies to endomysium (EMA) and gliadin (AGA). Ab determination as screening for untreated CD

	Flat mucosa		Normal mucosa	
EMA +				
⎧ IgG AND IgA-AGA +	247/248	99.6%	1/248	(0.4%)
⎨ IgG-AGA +, IgA-AGA –	56/58	(96.4%)	2/58	(0.6%)
⎩ No AGA	1/2		1/2	
EMA –				
⎧ IgG and IgA-AGA +	24/35	(68%)	11/35	(32%)
⎨ IgG-AGA +, IgA-AGA –	8/68	(12%)	60/68	(88%)
⎩ No AGA	1/137	(0.7%)	136/137	99.3%

137 or 99.3% of patients with neither gliadin nor endomysium ab had a normal mucosa. Conversely, the percentage of patients with normal mucosae decreases if one, two or even three tests are positive. Of a total of 548 biopsied patients with gliadin and endomysium ab determinations, 385 or 70% had three concordant ab results. The question could now be discussed whether it would not be possible to refrain from carrying out biopsies in these two groups of patients with three concordant tests. The chance of an incorrect result is extremely small. In general, a positive antibody test for coeliac disease indicates the necessity for a small bowel biopsy. Conversely, a negative response for all three antibodies indicates that a biopsy is not required, if the patient is younger than two years of age and is not IgA deficient. But, instead of performing first and second biopsies which do not exclude transient coeliac disease, especially in children

younger than two years old, we could set up other diagnostic criteria. These could include clinical symptoms and gliadin and EMA ab determinations, followed by clinical and serological responses after withdrawal of gluten from the diet. This would certainly demand a challenge followed by a biopsy. This final biopsy, after challenge, would give a definitive answer as to whether a patient is suffering from persistent CD. In our studies, we have 15 correctly diagnosed patients without relapse after 4–15 years of gliadin intake. This proposal for one biopsy at the end of the diagnostic procedure, instead of three biopsies or of one at the beginning, recently proposed by Guandalini et al.[20], is contrary to the generally accepted ESPGAN criteria[21]. In addition, three of the co-authors (H. Gaze, M. Lentze, and D. Nusslé) of this article still adhere to the ESPGAN dogma.

Ab determinations as a control of gluten-free diet

There is a rapid decrease of IgA gliadin ab, a slower decrease of endomysium ab and a very slow decrease of IgG gliadin ab. Therefore, during the first months on a gliadin-free diet the IgA gliadin ab test is most useful. After one or more years of diet, all tests should be negative.

Ab determinations as a control of persistent gluten intolerance

Ab to *gliadin* appear *earlier* after challenge than ab to endomysium. Therefore, after a *short-time* challenge, antigliadin ab are *more sensitive*.

Antibodies to *endomysium are more sensitive* for the detection of silent relapse after *prolonged periods of gluten intake*.

A combination of both tests gives best results. In only 3/124 patients with relapse, could no antibodies be found.

Acknowledgements

For enabling me to speak about the diagnostic significance of gliadin and endomysium ab, I should like to express my cordial thanks to the numerous gastroenterologists in Switzerland and Germany who sent me the clinical reports on their patients. I especially want to thank Prof Shmerling from Zürich, Prof K. Harms and Dr R. Bertele-Harms from Munich, and Dr Reymond who wrote her thesis on endomysium ab. And also all the other gastroenterologists who have helped me to collect data on so many patients with jejunal biopsy.

References

1. Berger, E. (1958). *Zur Allergischen Pathogenese der Cöliakie. Aus dem Kinderspital Basel.* (Basel: Verlag S. Karger)
2. Bürgin-Wolff, A., Hernandez, R. and Just, M. (1972). A rapid fluorescent solid-phase

method for detecting antibodies against milk proteins and gliadin in different immunoglobulin classes. *Experientia,* **28**, 119–120

3. Bürgin-Wolff, A., Hernandez, R., Just, M. and Signer, E. (1976). Immunofluorescent antibodies against gliadin: a screening test for coeliac disease. *Helv. Paediatr. Acta,* **31**, 375–380

4. Bürgin-Wolff, A., Bertele, R.M., Berger, R., Gaze, H., Harms, H.K., Just, M., Khanna, S., Schürmann, K., Signer, E. and Tomivic, D. (1983). A reliable screening test for childhood celiac antibodies. *J Pediatr.,* **102**, 655–660

5. Bürgin-Wolff, A., Berger, R., Gaze, H., Lentze, M.J. and Nusslé, D. (1989). IgG, IgA and IgE gliadin antibody determinations as screening test for untreated coeliac disease in children, a multicenter study. *Eur. J. Pediatr.,* **148**, 496–502

6. Signer, E., Bürgin-Wolff, A., Berger, R., Birbaumer, A. and Just, M. (1979). Antibodies to gliadin as a screening test for coeliac disease. *Helv. Paediatr. Acta,* **34**, 41–52

7. Blazer, S., Naveh, Y., Berant, M., Merzbach, D. and Sperber, S. (1984). Serum IgG antibodies to gliadin in children with celiac disease as measured by an immunofluorescence method. *J. Pediatr. Gastroenterol. Nutr.,* **3**, 205–209

8. Granditsch, G. (1983). Der Nachweis von Antikörpern gegen Gliadin im Serum mittels Enzymimmunoassay und indirekter Immunfluoreszenz und seine Bedeutung für die Diagnostik der Coeliakie im Kindesalter. *Wien. Klin. Wochenschr. (Suppl.),* **140**, 1–48

9. Juto, P., Fredrikzon, B. and Hernell, O. (1985). Gliadin-specific serum immunoglobulins A, E, G, and M in childhood: relation to small intestine mucosal morphology. *J. Pediatr. Gastroenterol. Nutr.,* **4**, 723–729

10. Kelly, J., O'Farrelly, C., Rees, J.P.R., Feighery, C. and Weir, D.G.W. (1987). Humoral response to alpha gliadin as serological screening test for coeliac disease. *Arch. Dis. Child.,* **62**, 469–473

11. Kieffer, M. (1985). Serum antibodies to gliadin and other cereal proteins in patients with coeliac disease and dermatitis herpetiformis. *Dan. Med. Bull.,* **32**, 251–262

12. Koninckx, C.R., Giliams, J.P., Polanco, I. and Peña, A.S. (1984). IgA antigliadin antibodies in celiac and inflammatory bowel disease. *J. Pediatr. Gastroenterol. Nutr.,* **3**, 676–682

13. Savilahti, E., Perkkiö, M., Kalimo, K., Viander, M., Vainio, E. and Reunala, T. (1983). IgA antigliadin antibodies: a marker of mucosal damage in childhood coeliac disease. *Lancet,* **1**, 320–322

14. Scott, H., Fausa, O., Ek, J. and Brandtzaeg, P. (1984). Immune response patterns in coeliac disease. Serum antibodies to dietary antigens measured by an enzyme linked immunosorbent assay (ELISA). *Clin. Exp. Immunol.,* **57**, 25–32

15. Stenhammar, L., Kilander, A.F., Nilsson, L.A., Strömberg, L. and Tarkowski, A. (1984). Serum gliadin antibodies for detection and control of childhood coeliac disease. *Acta Paediatr. Scand.,* **73**, 657–663

16. Troncone, R., Pignata, C., Farris, E. and Ciccimarra, F. (1983). A solid-phase radioimmunoassay for IgG gliadin antibodies using 125 I-labelled staphylococcal protein A. *J. Immunol. Meth.,* **63**, 163–170

17. Volta, U., Lenzi, M., Lazzari, R., Cassani, F., Collina, A., Bianchi, F.B. and Pisi, E. (1985). Antibodies to gliadin detected by immunofluorescence and a micro-ELISA method: markers of active childhood and adult coeliac disease. *Gut,* **26**, 667–671

18. Chorzelski, T.P., Sulej, J., Tchorzewska, H., Jablonska, S., Beutner, E.H. and Kumar, V. (1983). IgA class endomysium antibodies (IgA-EMA) in dermatitis herpetiformis and coeliac disease. *Ann. N.Y. Acad. Sci.,* **420**, 324–325

19. Chorzelski, T.P., Jablonska, S., Beutner, E.H., Kumar, V., Sulej, J. and Leonard, J.N. (1987). Anti-endomysial antibodies in dermatitis herpetiformis and celiac disease. In Beutner, E.H., Chorzelski, T.P. and Kumar, V. (eds.) *Immunopathology of the Skin,* 3rd edn., pp. 477–482 (New York: Wiley)

20. Guandalini, S., Ventura, A., Ansaldi, N., Giunta, A.M., Greco, L., Lazzari, R., Mastella, G. and Rubino, A. (1989). Diagnosis of coeliac disease: time for a change? *Arch. Dis. Child.,* **64**, 1320–1325

21. McNeish, A.S., Harms, H.K., Rey, J., Shmerling, D.H., Visakorpi, J.K. and Walker-Smith, J.A. (1979). The diagnosis of coeliac disease. *Arch. Dis. Child.,* **54**, 783–786

17
Concluding remarks

F. HADZISELIMOVIC

After two days of intensive and fruitful work, we have reached the end of the First International Symposium on Inflammatory Bowel Disease and Coeliac Disease. On this occasion, I would like to express the thanks of all participants to Dr Falk for making this meeting possible. I would also like to thank Hoffmann-La Roche Company for sharing their facilities with us.

This meeting has stressed again the importance of a joint venture between paediatricians and paediatric surgeons in addressing a common problem. The theme of this symposium was not chosen without considerable deliberation.

The aetiology of inflammatory bowel disease (IBD) is still unknown despite intensive scientific research during recent years. It was nicely shown yesterday that the gut, an organ of 300 m^2 surface, is also a major immunological contact organ. The mucosa enables controlled antigen uptake. Mucosal development reaches its maximum size during the first year and remains constant thereafter. Additional research will determine whether environmental influences and a modified diet play an important role during the early development of the mucosa. These factors may be responsible for the increased incidence in recent years of Crohn's disease (CD).

CD appears to be an inherited disease, more so than ulcerative colitis. For example, there is increased familial incidence, different frequency of incidence among different ethnic groups, and association of CD with other diseases that have no genetic predispositions. However, genetic factors need additional stimuli in order for CD to develop. Smoking habits and the use of the contraceptive pill have been implicated as important mediators of the disease. Last week, in their feature article in *The Lancet*, Wakefield *et al.* suggested[1] that these two potentially thrombogenic agents may augment disease activity by exacerbating underlying vesicular injury and tendency to focal thrombosis. Interestingly enough, smoking seemed to determine the type of IBD in genetically predisposed individuals.

Since the gut is the largest immune organ of the body, it is not surprising that disequilibrium in the immune system has been claimed as an aetiological factor of IBD:

(1) CD patients with colonic inflammation had a significantly higher subset of lymphocytes with TCR_1 receptors compared with normal individuals.

(2) Also, CD patients with an $A_{10}-B_{18}$ HLA haplotype had an inherited C_2 complement deficiency which is usually associated with IBD.

(3) CD patients and their relatives had a significantly greater ADCC (antibody dependent cellular cytotoxicity). Responsiveness that can be interpreted as an inherited aberrant immunological phenomenon rather than a response to specific viral antigens. However, an environmental cause for the increased titre of immunoglobulin cannot be disregarded.

Ulcerative colitis (UC), on the other hand, is likely to develop in children under 10 years of age. Pathogenesis leading to the mucosal damage is still unknown; however, the process, once initiated, seems to be self-perpetuating. There is ample evidence that alterations in the immune system may be responsible. Pronounced infiltration of lamina propria with plasma cells supports this hypothesis. A constant local irritation of gut mucosa may, however, lead to breakdown in the second line of defense in the gut which results in ulcerative colitis.

We have learned that efficacy of endoscopy as a diagnostic procedure is as high as 94% with diagnostic specificity of 84%. Furthermore, 40% of patients endoscopically examined had positive histological but negative radiological findings. Unfortunately, there is not a single endoscopical, radiological or clinical parameter that is able to distinguish specifically between CD and UC. Furthermore, we have absolutely no specific histological parameter today that enables us to distinguish between CD and UC.

Therefore, computer tomography and ultrasound are important additional aids in the diagnostic evaluation of patients with IBD. This is particularly relevant in that early diagnosis is extremely important and that only 22% of patients are diagnosed correctly by attending physicians at the time of admission (see B. Kirshner, this volume). Growth retardation is a specific paediatric problem, predominantly found in CD. Somatomedin-C levels were low in growth-impaired children with IBD. Significant correlation was found to exist between somatomedin-C levels and nutritional status as well as growth velocity. The question to be answered in the near future is whether the determination of growth hormone in urine can be used as a disease-activity parameter in patients with IBD. The treatment of IBD requires the collaborative effort of paediatric gastroenterologists, paediatric surgeons, paediatric radiologists and paediatric endocrinologists. Competent psychological support for the entire family of chronically ill children is also an important consideration. Medical treatment primarily consists of corticosteroids and sulphosalazine as well as hyperalimentation. In males, however, sulphosalazine induces testicular changes at the level of late spermatids which can result in infertility unless remedial action is taken. 5-ASA has been shown to have fewer side-effects in adults. Its efficacy in children seems to be as high as sulphosalazine. The use of sugar-free diet in patients with CD is still controversial today. More work needs to be done before a general consensus can be reached.

Nearly all patients with severe UC and at least 70% of patients with CD will ultimately require surgery. It is clear and unanimous that surgery for IBD should be elective and optimally timed. In patients with CD, it should be kept to a minimum, while, in patients with UC, it should be radical. The excellent collaboration between surgeons and internists is an absolute prerequisite for optimal treatment of these children.

Grain prolamins are essential in the aetiology of coeliac disease. 13 mg/day for a period of 10 years seems to be tolerated in children with coeliac disease. An important conclusion to be drawn today is that 10 mg gliadin seems to be the upper limit of non-toxic effect. However, gliadin is immunogenic, not only in coeliac patients, but also in patients having greater permeability in the upper gastrointestinal tract and, to a lesser extent, in normal individuals. This immunogenicity stems from poor digestion and, perhaps, the structure of the protein itself. Although the aetiology of coeliac disease is still a mystery, we have made significant progress in the diagnosis of coeliac disease during the past 20 years. It seems appropriate to mention Professor Berger's research in our hospital here in Basel (see Bürgin-Wolff et al., this volume) . Twenty-seven years ago, he was the first to draw attention to the elevated gliadin antibodies in patients with coeliac disease. Combined determination of gliadin and endomysium antibodies has proved to have important diagnostic significance. Almost 100% of children with coeliac disease were positive for the combined test. With the help of this diagnostic test, our institution has abolished the second biopsy. Whether the first biopsy should be performed depends, not only on the results of combined antibody tests, but also on the clinical status of the patient. It is the clinician who is ultimately responsible for deciding whether the biopsy should be obtained or not, since each patient expresses the clinical features differently.

Although there has been a strong tendency at this meeting to distinguish coeliac disease as a unique and separate disease, nevertheless, all three inflammatory diseases of the gut, M. Crohn, UC, and coeliac disease, have been associated with each other.

For example, the courses of UC and coeliac disease of the large bowel are totally similar to each other with both being different from coeliac disease of the small bowel. A. Logan[2] has recently reported that changing environmental factors, such as smoking, can mediate changes in expression of IBD from Crohn's disease to ulcerative colitis. Ulcerative colitis has been shown to appear more often in patients with coeliac disease than in their relatives as compared with the control population[3].

Crohn's disease was also found in patients with coeliac disease, and the existence of gliadin antibodies in patients with Crohn's disease provides additional evidence for the link between these two diseases.

Intestinal permeability for [^{51}Cr]EDTA is increased among children with Crohn's disease or coeliac disease[4]. Furthermore, transcellular uptake of mannitol is affected in both Crohn's and coeliac diseases[5] and local release of neutrophil and eosinophil granule components is enhanced in the jejunal tissue from patients with coeliac and Crohn's disease[6].

It is obvious that all three diseases have demonstrated an intimate involvement of the immune system as a predominant feature. T-suppressor cell defect was described in all three disease[7-10].

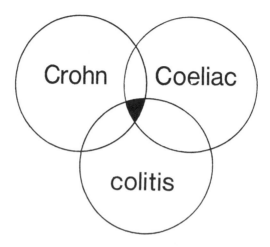

Figure 1 CCC disease

Ample evidence has been presented during the past two days to support the hypothesis for a combined CCC disease (Crohn–Colitis–Coeliac disease; Figure 1) as an inflammatory bowel disease with different expression of a genetically determined inflammation of the bowel. It remains to be seen in the future whether this model will stand the test of time.

References

1. Wakefield, A.J., Sawyerr, A.M., Dhillon, A.P., Pittilo, R.M., Rowles, P.M., Lewis, A.A.M. and Pounder, R.E. (1989). Pathogenesis of Crohn's disease: multifocal gastrointestinal infarction. *Lancet*, **2**, 1057–1062
2. Logan, R.F.A. (1988). Smoking and inflammatory bowel disease. In Goebell, H., Peskar, B.M. and Malchow, H. (eds.) *Inflammatory Bowel Diseases*, pp. 215–223 (Lancaster: MTP Press Limited)
3. Peña, A.S. (1990). Genetics of inflammatory bowel disease. This volume, Chap. 2
4. Turck, D., Ythier, H., Maquet, E., Deveaux, M., Marchandise, X., Farriaux, J.P. and Fontaine, G. (1987). Intestinal permeability to [51Cr]EDTA in children with Crohn's disease and celiac disease. *J. Pediatr. Gastroenterol. Nutr.*, **6**, 535–537
5. Dawson, D.J., Lobley, R.W., Burrows, P.C., Notman, J.A., Mahon, M. and Holmes, R. (1988). Changes in jejunal permeability and passive permeation of sugars in intestinal biopsies in coeliac disease and Crohn's disease. *Clin. Sci.*, **742**, 427–431
6. Hällgren, R., Colombel, J.F., Dahl, R., Fredens, K., Kruse, A., Jacobsen, N.O., Venge, P. and Rambaud, J.C. (1989). Neutrophil and eosinophil involvement of the small bowel in patients with celiac disease and Crohn's disease: studies in the secretion rate and immunohistochemical localization of granulocyte granule constitutents. *Am. J. Med.*, **68**, 56–64
7. Strober, W. and James, S.P. (1986). The immunologic basis of inflammatory bowel disease. *J. Clin. Immunol.*, **6**, 415

8. Soppi, E., Eskola, J., Lehtonen, O.-P. and Leino, R. (1988). Immune functions in inflammatory bowel and coeliac diseases. *Acta Pathol. Microbiol. Scand.,* **96**, 850–856
9. Seidman, E., Morin, C.L., Weber, A.M., Lenaerts, C. and Roy, C.C. (1989). Inflammatory bowel disease in children. In Freeman, H.J. (ed.) *Inflammatory Bowel Disease*, Vol. II (Boca Raton, Florida: CRC Press Inc.)
10. Walker-Smith, J.A. (1990). Management of coeliac disease in children: a personal view. This volume, Chap. 13

Index

adrenoreceptors, lymphocyte 36
ankylosing spondylitis, IBD
 association 49, 52
anorectal lesions 119
antigen degradation 13, 14
antigen uptake 13–21, 22
 age-dependent 17–20
 decrease, IgA antibody-associated 20
 increase, disease-associated 21
antigens, oral tolerance 3
appendix vermiformis 4, 30–1
 lymphatic follicles 31
 lymphatic tissue, postnatal
  development 32–5
5-ASA (mesalazine) 190
 azathioprine combination, UC 90, 91
 IBD 87–8, 89–96
 nephrotoxicity 88
 ulcerative colitis 88, 90, 91
atopic eczema
 IBD association 50
 intestinal permeability 21
autoimmune disease, IBD association 50
azathioprine
 IBD 89, 90
 mesalazine combination, UC 90, 91

bacterial counts
 GI tract 4–5
 see also microbial status
Best index 93
breast milk, antibody content 19–20
brush (striated) border 7, 9

caloric insufficiency, childhood IBD 62
CCC disease 191–2
CD3⁺CD4⁻CD8⁻ cells, coeliac
 disease 150–1
CD4:CD8 T cell ratio, follicle-associated
 epithelium 24
children, Crohn's disease see paediatric
 Crohn's disease
children, IBD 59–65
 aetiopathogenesis 59–60
 clinical diversity 60–3
 diagnostic imaging 75–82
 endocrine studies 62–3
 epidemiology 59
 extraintestinal manifestations 60–1

growth failure 61–3
 reversal 63
 intestinal involvement 60
 surgery 117–20
children, ulcerative colitis 59–65
 Crohn's disease differentiation 78, 80
 diagnostic imaging 75–8
chromatid bodies, SASP effects 99–111
circulating antibodies, coeliac disease 152,
 153
 see also endomysium antibodies; gliadin
  antibodies
coeliac disease
 circulating antibodies 152, 153
 control, antibody determination 186
 diagnostic biopsy analysis 149
 diagnostic criteria 147–8
 endomysium antibodies 177–87
 gliadin antibodies 164, 165, 177–87
 gluten-free diet
  antibodies 181–2
  duration 153–4
 HLA association 169–73, 174
 IBD association 50
 IgE antibodies 179–80
 IgG/IgA gliadin antibodies 179
 intestinal permeability 21
 intraepithelial lymphocyte
  analysis 149–51
 management 147–55
 screening, antibody determination 183,
  185–6
colectomy, total, ileorectostomy 124, 125,
 126
colonic surface epithelium 7
colorectal cancer risk, Crohn's disease 55
columnar villous epithelium 7
complement allotypes, susceptibility
 markers 52
computerized tomography (CT), ulcerative
 colitis 75–8
continent ileostomy (Kock pouch) 124,
 125–6, 127, 128
contraceptive pill, Crohn's disease 54, 55
cow's milk-sensitive enteropathy 149
Crohn's disease
 abnormal bacterial flora 53
 activity indices (PCDAIs) 93–6
 ankylosing spondylitis 49, 52

Crohn's disease (*continued*)
  azathioprine 89
  colorectal cancer risk 55
  complement allotypes 52
  conservative treatment, flow sheet 96, 97
  contraceptive pill 54, 55
  familial aspects 46, 189
  genetic aspects 45–58
  growth failure, surgery 118
  ileal permeability 21
  intestinal permeability increase 53
  lymphocyte subsets 83–6
  and M cells 15
  metronidazole 89
  sarcoidosis association 51
  semi-elemental diet 92–3
  SLE 50
  spouses 46, 48
  surgery, indications 118, 120
  see also paediatric Crohn's disease
crypt epithelium 10, 11
crypts of Lieberkuhn 7

dermatitis herpetiformis 177
desmosomes 10

endomysium antibodies
  coeliac disease 177–87
  determination 178
  gluten challenge 182–3, 185
endoscopic diagnostic criteria, Crohn's
  disease 68, 69
endoscopic lesions, Crohn's disease
  classification 68
  diagnostic sensitivities 71–2, 73
  frequencies 71
  location 69–71
endoscopy, IBD 190
enterocytes, particle uptake 14–15
environmental factors 54–5
epithelium
  follicle-associated 15, 16, 17, 18
    bidirectional transport 21
    CD4:CD8 ratio 24
    T cells 23–4
  kinetics 10, 12–13
  life cycle, gut microbial status 12–13
  lymphocytes 22–5
  structures 7–10, 11, 12
ESPGAN (Interlaken) criteria, coeliac
  disease 147–8
ethnic groups, IBD incidence 46, 49

faecal continence preservation, UC
  surgery 123–5
food allergy, secretory Ig deficiencies 34
FSH, plasma levels, SASP effects 103, 113

germinal centres 4
Giardia lamblia, M cell penetration 15
glandulae intestinalis 7
gliadin
  immunogenicity 157–67, 191
  toxic levels 164, 165
  types 159
gliadin antibodies
  age group levels 157–8, 159
  coeliac disease 152, 153, 164, 165, 177–87
  determination 178
  gluten challenge 182, 183, 184
  immunocrossreactivity 160–4
gluten challenge
  coeliac disease 148–9
  emdomysium antibodies 182–3, 185
  gliadin antibodies 182, 183, 184
  indications 148–9
  technique 153–4
gluten intolerance
  persistent
    antibody determination 186
    see also coeliac disease
  transient 151–2
gluten-free diet, coeliac disease
  antibodies 181–2
  control, antibody determination 186
  duration 153–4
glycocalyx 9
glycogen storage disease type Ib (GSB-Ib),
  and Crohn's disease 51
glycoproteins, colonic 54
growth failure, childhood IBD
  mechanisms 61–2
  reversal 63
growth hormone (GH), childhood IBD 62
gut
  antigenic burden 4–5
  as immunologic organ 3
gut-associated lymphoid tissue
  (GALT) 3–4, 29–31
  postnatal development/maintenance
    32–5

Hashimoto's disease, ulcerative colitis 50
histocompatibility antigens (HLA),
  susceptibility markers 52
HLA-B27, ankylosing spondylitis, IBD 49, 50
HLA-B8/DR3, primary sclerosing
  cholangitis 51
HLA-complex 169–70
  class II molecules 170–2
  small intestine 172–3
HLA-DQ, coeliac disease
  association 171–2, 174

HLA-DR
  coeliac disease association 170-2
  enterocyte antigen uptake 12, 13, 14
HLA-DR-like antigens 10, 12

IgA
  intestinal, precursor cell
    stimulation/circulation 27
  mucosal lamina propria 25, 26, 27
IgA antibodies
  antigen uptake reduction 20
  breast milk 19-20
  gliadin, coeliac disease 179
IgE antibodies, gliadin, coeliac
    disease 179-80
IgG antibodies, gliadin, coeliac disease 179
ileoanal anastomoses 124
ileoanal endorectal pullthrough
  advantages/disadvantages 127, 128
  complications 126, 127
ileorectostomy 124, 125, 126
  advantages/disadvantages 127, 128
ileostomy
  continent (Kock pouch) 124, 125-6, 127,
    128
  ulcerative colitis 123-8
immune disequilibrium, IBD 189-90
immunocrossreactivity, prolamins 160-4
immunocytes, as endocrine cells 35-6
immunoglobulin allotypes, susceptibility
    markers 52
immunological contact sites 15
infertility, male, sulphasalazine-related
    99-106
inflammatory bowel disease (IBD)
  aetiology 189-90
  associated diseases 49-51
  familial aggregations 45-6
  medical treatment 63, 87-98
  see also children, IBD; Crohn's disease;
    ulcerative colitis
interleukins 36
intestinal absorption, growth failure and
    IBD 61
intestinal mucosa, flat, coeliac disease 147,
    149
intestinal permeability, increased, Crohn's
    disease 53
intra-/interpersonal factors, in IBD
    aetiology 137-8
intraepithelial lymphocytes 22-5
  coelic disease 149-51
  T-cell lymphocytes 24-5

junctional complex, epithelial cell 10

Kallman's syndrome, ulcerative colitis
    association 51
Kerckring's folds 7

Kock continent ileostomy 124, 125-6, 127
  advantages/disadvantages 127, 128

β-lactoglobulin antibodies 157, 158
lamina propria, mucosal, as lymphoid
    organ 25-9
LH, plasma levels, SASP effects 103, 112
Lieberkuhn's crypts 7
lupus erythematosus, systemic (SLE)
  HLA-DR2 association 52
  IBD association 50
lymphatic follicles 4
  neonatal appendix 32, 33
  Peyer's patches 29-30
  plasma cells 30
  solitary 30, 31
  vermiform appendix 31
  zones 29
lymphocytes
  adrenoreceptors 36
  intraepithelial 22-5
    coeliac disease 149-51
    T cell lymphocytes 24-5
lymphocytotoxic antibodies (LCA),
    susceptibility markers 53
M cells 15
  as infection channels 15, 17, 19, 20
macrophages, intraepithelial lymphocyte
    contact 28-9
macula adherens 10
mesalazine (5-ASA) 190
  azathioprine combination, UC 90, 91
  IBD 87-8, 86-96
  nephrotoxicity 88
  ulcerative colitis 88
mesenteric lymph nodes 30
metronidazole, Crohn's disease 89
microbial status, intestinal 12-13
microvilli 7, 8
migrants, IBD incidence 49
Mikulicz spur, terminal ileum/sigmoid
    colon 123
mucin species IV deficiency, ulcerative
    colitis 54
mucosal block, gut antigens 3, 5-13
mucosal immune system 26-8
mucosal stripping, transanal 124
mucus layer 6-7
multiple sclerosis, IBD association 50

neonates, gut antigen absorption 17-20
neuroimmunoendocrinology 35-6
neurotic traits, and IBD 139-40
nuclear lysis, spermatid/spermatocyte,
    SASP-related 102, 107
paediatric Crohn's disease 59-65
  activity indices (PCDAIs) 93-6
  age distribution 69

paediatric Crohn's disease (*continued*)
  barium studies 78, 79, 81
  CD3⁺CD4⁻CD8⁻ cells 83-6
  computerized tomography 78, 79
  diagnostic sensitivities 71-2
  endoscopic evaluation 67-74
  height velocity 134, 135
  lymphocyte subsets 83-6
  postoperative recurrence 119, 131-6
    anatomical location effects 132, 133
  postoperative recurrence and resection
    indication 132, 133, 134
  UC differentiation 78, 80
  ultrasound scans 78, 81
Paneth cells 10
PCDAIs 93-6
perineal lesions 119
Peyer's patches 29
  and microbial status 13
  structure 29, 30
phagolysosomes 13
plasma cells
  IgA secretion 25, 26, 27
  neonatal appendix 32-3, 34
plicae circulares 7
prednisone, IBD 87, 90
premature infants, alimentary antigen
    uptake 17-19
primary sclerosing cholangitis (PSC), IBD
    association 50-1
proctocolectomy
  ileostomy 122-3, 125, 126
    advantages/disadvantages 127, 128
  ulcerative colitis 119
prolamins
  grain 159-64
  immunocrossreactivity 160-4
  immunogenicity 157-67, 191
  see also endomysium; gliadin
protein status, childhood IBD 61
proteins, intestinal wall transport 157
pseudopolyposis, inflammatory, UC 91, 92
psoriasis, IBD association 49-50
psyche, and IBD 137-43
psychiatric disease, and IBD 139-40
psychosomatic aspects 137-43
psychotherapy, and IBD 140-3
pyomelanocortin (POMC) 35

regulatory factors, epithelial kinetics 10, 13
rheumatoid arthritis, intestinal
    permeability 21

sarcoidosis, Crohn's disease association 51
semi-elemental diet, Crohn's disease 92-3
SLE
  HLA-DR2 association 52
  IBD association 50

somatomedin-C 190
  childhood IBD 62
spermatids, nuclear degeneration,
    SASP-related 99-111
spermatocytes, nuclear degeneration, SASP
    effects 99-111
spermatogenesis, SASP effects 100, 101-11
spouses
  Crohn's disease 46, 48
  ulcerative colitis 46, 47
stress management therapy 141
stressful life events, and IBD 138-9
sulphapyridine, IBD 87, 88
sulphasalazine (SASP) 190-1
  androspermatozoides toxicity 101
  dosage/body weight 99, 100
  IBD 87-96
  prepubertal testes effects 99-115
  side-effects 98
  surgery 191
    emergency, prognosis 117
    indications 117, 118
    paediatric IBD 117-20
systemic lupus erythematosus (SLE)
  HLA-DR2 association 52
  IBD association 50

T-cell receptors
  coeliac disease 150-1
  intraepithelial lymphocytes 23, 24-5
T lymphocytes, antigen receptors 83-6
TCR1
  CD3⁺CD4⁻CD8⁻ cells 83-6
  paediatric Crohn's disease 83-6
TCR2 83
testes
  sulphasalazine effects 99-115
  weight, SASP effects 103, 115
testosterone, plasma/intratesticular, SASP
    effects 103, 114-15
thyroid function, childhood IBD 62
transanal mucosal stripping 124
transient gluten intolerance 151-2
trophic factors, epithelial kinetics 10
Turcot's syndrome 51
Turner syndrome, IBD association 51
twins, monozygous, IBD 46

ulcerative colitis
  genetic aspects 45-58
  mesalazine (5-ASA) 88
  mucin species IV deficiency 54
  prednisone 90
  spouses 46, 47
  surgery 121-9
    historical aspects 121-3
    indications 118, 120
ulcerative colitis, children 59-65

Crohn's disease differentiation 78, 80
    diagnostic imaging 75-8

van Hees index 93
'vascular addressin', lymphocyte 28
Vibrio cholerae, M cells 15

villi intestinalis 7
villous atrophy, hyperplastic, coeliac
    disease 147-8

zona occludens 10
zonula adherens 10